Cooking Well

Multiple Sclerosis

Chef Marie-Annick Courtier

Dedication

I dedicate this book to my friends, Susie and Jackie, who have both been diagnosed with Multiple Sclerosis.

—Chef Marie

COOKING WELL. MULTIPLE SCLEROSIS

www.hatherleighpress.com

DISCLAIMER
This book offers healthy eating suggestions for educational purposes only. In no case should it be a substitute for, nor replace, a healthcare professional. Consult your healthcare professional before starting any new diet.

Library of Congress Cataloging-in-Publication Data

Courtier, Marie-Annick.
Cooking well. Multiple sclerosis / Marie-Annick Courtier.
p. cm.
Includes bibliographical references.

ISBN 978-1-57826-301-1 (pbk. : alk. paper) 1. Multiple sclerosis—Diet therapy—Recipes. 2. Low-fat diet—Recipes. 3. Inflammation—Diet therapy—Recipes. I. Title. II. Title: Multiple sclerosis.
RC377.C678 2009
641.5'638—dc22

2009010621

Cover design by Nick Macagnone
Photo by Catarina Astrom
10 9 8 7 6 5 4 3 2 1

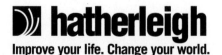

We have long known that proper nutrition plays an important role in guarding health and preventing the onset of disease. The *Cooking Well* series was created to help you learn more about the important role of nutrient-rich meals when living with your particular disorder. With *Cooking Well*, you will discover that there are many enjoyable ways to prepare delightful, great-tasting meals that are packed with a variety of healthful benefits.

Chef Marie-Annick Courtier, a well-known culinary and health expert, has utilized her background in nutrition and health studies to create easy to prepare meals that are good for you and so delicious that you and your entire family can enjoy them together. Chef Marie was born in Paris, where she acquired a knowledge of fresh, flavorful food that she incorporates into her healthy recipes. Today, Chef Marie is a widely-published author who also owns and operates a personal chef service.

Hatherleigh has a long history of providing our readers with books that help people improve their lives, whether through exercise, nutrition, or mental well-being. We are pleased to share with you the message of good health in the *Cooking Well* series.

—*Andrew Flach, Publisher*

Table of Contents

Foreword

As a doctor and patient with Multiple Sclerosis, I am familiar with the day to day challenge of managing this condition and keeping up with the latest news on treatment. We've come so far since 1990, when there were no therapies available to alter the course of Multiple Sclerosis. Currently, we have six therapies to slow down MS and six more that are in either clinical or pre-clinical testing (including two oral medications). This is wonderful news.

However, those of us who have MS know that, because MS abuses our brains and spinal cords, we must do everything we can to keep our bodies in the best shape possible. We routinely go to physical, occupational and cognitive therapies and attend informational meetings and support groups. Yet one aspect of therapy that we commonly overlook is eating well.

Many of us know that we should eat foods that are rich in fiber and protein, and that we should avoid saturated fats and cholesterol. But, on a day to day basis, our meals are often lacking. It can seem daunting to prepare healthy meals several times each day, so we tend to stop trying. After awhile, we come to believe that we simply don't have enough time or energy to devote to a proper diet.

I know we can do better. The recipes in this book will open your eyes to how easy and fun it can be to maintain a balanced diet. With the fresh, healthful ingredients in these appetizing meals, you will provide your body with the nutrients it needs to keep you healthy. Diet can be an effective therapy for guarding your health, and it's time to make it a priority.

I feel it is our duty as patients with MS to make sure that we keep our bodies in the best shape possible while the doctors and scientists continue to work toward the ultimate goal for our disease—the cure.

Vincent F. Macaluso, MD
5/14/09

Part I

Understanding Multiple Sclerosis

Chapter 1

Living with Multiple Sclerosis

Multiple Sclerosis (MS) is an inflammatory demyelinating disorder of the human central nervous system (CNS). It is a progressive disease from which 2.5 million people in the world suffer, about 400,000 of whom live in the United States. This number is increasing by 200 people monthly. The disease is much more common among women and its impact on family life can be very devastating. Symptoms vary from weakness, spasticity (tightness), balance problems, bladder problems, slurred speech, pain, fatigue, cognitive problems, numbness, and blurred vision. Practicing a healthy lifestyle has shown to help many patients with MS. Exercising regularly, reducing stress, not smoking, learning about yourself and your limits, maintaining a healthy weight, and eating a healthy diet are crucial for better well-being.

As of today, there is actually no specific scientific data or studies done on any specific diet for MS patients. However, **many people report major improvements in their well-being once they change their eating habits.** Identifying individual food sensitivities and allergies plays an important role and designing the right diet for each individual is primordial. In the last few years, a significant collection of information on eating habits for people suffering from MS has the medical corps rethinking the importance of diet. It is possible that certain foods may even contribute to causing MS or increasing its symptoms. A list of specific foods to avoid has emerged, as many people have reported improvement after eliminating them from their diet. Other diseases, such as Celiac Disease, call for avoiding similar foods. In many cases, people reported decrease of symptoms, flare-ups and, for some, even almost complete relief from MS symptoms, allowing them to live a normal life as long as they maintained a healthy lifestyle. Eating a low fat diet with foods high in anti-inflammatory properties seems to have helped many people with MS. Consequently, this will be the focus of this book.

Lifestyle

Many people struggling with diseases, weight problems, or allergies, often don't make the connection between their eating habits and their lifestyle choices. They often do not realize how much their emotions influence everything they do in their life, including the food they eat or finding excuses not to exercise. Unfortunately those emotions can trigger eating habits that will be the cause for more pain, worse symptoms, and be very detrimental to their health.

Consequently, **it is imperative that each individual look into his or her lifestyle and emotions to see how they affect food choices.** It is recommended that you do this with your physician, registered dietitian, psychologist, or care giver.

MS patients should not smoke, as tobacco negatively impacts many organs of the body and is the leading cause for lung cancer. If you do smoke and have trouble quitting, consult your physician and psychologist. Here are a few tricks to get you started on improving your health. Start by looking into your daily routine to determine what may cause bad eating habits. For example: Do you eat a bunch of pastries or donuts in the morning, knowing you should have a more balanced breakfast? Do you often skip lunch, not feeling like eating? Do you snack all day and, consequently, are not hungry for a healthy dinner? Do you reach for the cookie jar when you are stressed? Do you drink soda when eating out? Those are just a few examples to get you thinking about what you do on a daily basis.

Chapter 2

How the Right Diet Can Help

Eating well can make a big difference in how you feel. But how should you begin to make a change, and how will you know what steps to take? Start to think about the time you felt well and when you started not to feel well. Review your journal to see what you did in the last 48 hours—what you ate, what you drank, if you ate out, over-exercised, worked too hard, skipped or change your medicine, or just went through treatment after a relapse. If you are no longer keeping a journal, it is time to start again. Can an emotional event or a stressful situation be triggering the problem? Is a situation making you irritable or frustrated? Are you anxious about a situation (moving or pregnancy)? Are you depressed for any reasons? Do you have sexual tension? Did you just introduce a new food into your diet? Did you go off your diet? Did you have a sleepless night or wake up many times for different reasons? Are you traveling or did you return from a vacation and resume work right away? Has the weather changed dramatically? Some patients have reported relapses a few days after weather changes. Beware and watch for seasonal changes, and try to relax more than usual during those times. Rest more by taking a one or two hour nap during those days (this is a good suggestion for any day you feel tired or somehow off.) Are you constipated to the point you are not feeling well? Sometimes the answer is right in front of you and a little thinking can elicit it.

Once you figure out your triggers, make sure you watch out for that situation in order to avoid repeating it. On the other hand, you might not discover right away t the reason for your crisis. You need to show patience, as it may take you awhile. A positive attitude and a strong will to determine why you are not feeling well is extremely important. Revise your strategies, goals, and any notes that you made for establishing your healthier lifestyle.

Remember, your goal is to live a better, healthier life with as few MS symptoms as possible.

If you avoid certain foods due to sensitivities or allergies, it is important to remember that you may deprive your body of major nutrients. This could be the reason why you do not feel well. Consult your physician or registered dietitian to see if you need to take vitamin and mineral supplementation. Review your diet with them carefully. If you have a caregiver, talk about your findings, as he/she can help you out as well.

A Word on Food Allergies and Sensitivities

As was mentioned earlier, determining your food allergies and sensitivities are extremely important. Consult your physician. One aspect a physician may not approach with you is the potential reasons behind those allergies or sensitivities. Our brain has many ways to tell us things or warn us. One of these is when an emotional event is attached to a particular food or scent, which can result in triggering a sudden allergy or sensitivity to that particular food or scent. The sensitivity does not necessarily surface at the time of the emotional event, but can be triggered later on in life. Our brain attaches the new event to the old event, and suddenly the allergy or sensitivity appears. Many events can be connected to the old event before something may even happen. Identifying those events in our lives can make a huge difference. Identifying the initial event in our lives that triggers the emotional chain will eventually lead to a breakthrough that may make the allergy or sensitivity disappear. The event can be related to our early childhood. Discuss this with your psychologist as he or she may be able to identify those moments, help you get over them and, consequently, eliminate certain allergies or food sensitivities. Be aware though that some allergies are truly immune system responses and are not connected to our emotions.

Talk to your family and friends. Take time to explain your diet to them and how it will benefit everyone, not just you. Tell them, if you get sick you will no longer be able to be involved in family and social activities, which you need for your own mental stability. However do not avoid your own responsibilities. You want to keep moving a bit to recover faster, so choose one chore you particularly enjoy. If you enjoy cooking, have everyone else do the prepping and cleaning, and choose easy, quick recipes that don't require much lifting and that are easy on your body. Such an attitude will make everyone much happier and less stressed, which is very important for MS patients and everyone else around them. Yes, it is about you, but also about everyone around you.

Let your caregiver, helpers, or family members know you need their support for the long run. Keep in mind that the comfort and kindness of a friend can go a long way and should be appreciated and treasured. You must remember to thank those who help you. Treat them with respect and even to a "special treat" once in awhile, as a small gesture can work wonders.

Do not feel intimidated to tell your friends what you can or cannot eat. They are your friends—they love you, and will understand. The last thing a real friend should do is not care for your health! **When you are feeling well, you can even write your own cook book with the foods that make you feel good and share it with your friends.** Read and educate yourself on MS. Read about the food that people with MS have reported helped them. See if it helps you as well.

Be aware that psychological and physical stress often results in fatigue, pains, and reduced abilities. One way to help you through difficult times of stress is through relaxation techniques and even mild exercises such as yoga. And don't forget about a nice refreshing bath, which can be very soothing. But be very cautious when entering and exiting the tub, to avoid falls, which often cause broken bones. Take some time off and pamper yourself!

Part II

The Importance of Nutrition

Chapter 3

Dietary Suggestions for a Healthy Lifestyle

No matter what your health problems, eating healthy foods should be a priority and a pleasant experience as well. You need to be responsible for your own health, don't expect anyone to keep you in line. As a matter of fact, many people will offer you foods that are not good for you and it is ultimately up to you to say "no, thank you." Pay particular attention to your nutrition plan and do everything in your power to stay as close to it as possible. You will feel much better, be able to enjoy your daily activities and reduce the risk of pains and, ultimately, of worsening your disease.

Eating habits are difficult to change and are often rooted in years of cultural and family habits. **Expecting a quick change is not realistic.** Patience and a strong will to change over time are a must. By employing new habits, you will eventually see the fruits of your labor in an improved overall well-being.

Healthy eating is not about eating everything you like. It is about giving your body what it needs and what agrees with it. It is about eating the right amount of calories per day considering your daily activities. Eating healthy is also about meal rituals. That means having regular meals at the same times every day. Three to four meals a day is recommended. That includes a snack in the afternoon, which is important to keep your blood sugar level stable if you have a late dinner. **It is ultimately up to you to decide what works best for your body and how to spread your meals throughout your day. Remember to appropriately divide your daily calories.** We will explore this further in the nutrition section when we specifically discuss which foods MS patients should eat and which they should avoid.

Eating Organic

Everyone knows that eating foods that are free of pesticides, chemicals, antibiotics, colorings, or hormones is better for you. This is strongly recommended for MS patients. If you are not financially strained, make an effort to shop organic at your local farmers' market, growers, and stores. If budget is an issue, do not stress about it. Sometimes we have to make practical decisions and, understandably, eating organic may not always be a priority. Also, keep in mind that due to very strict regulations, many farmers and growers are not able to obtain the organic label. But they are still producing foods that are free of pesticides, chemicals, antibiotics, and hormones, and are of excellent quality. All you need to do is find those products in your local stores and read their labels carefully.

Here are some buying tips that are economically prudent while also being healthier for you and your family. When buying dry, canned, or frozen products you should make sure to buy organic. They are not much more expensive and are much healthier for you. While you should not be eating such products on a regular basis, they can be helpful during the winter months, when a variety of vegetables and fruits are not available. Also if you cook for yourself and feel physically exhausted, you might opt for the dry, canned or frozen product.

Reduce your individual portions, particularly with meat products. You can stretch your dollars while you shrink your waistline. Portion sizes at your local store are often larger than what you really need to eat. For example, a chicken breast often weighs 8 ounces when you should only be eating about 4 ounces.

Support your local farmers and growers. The more distance the food travels from farm to table, the greater the cost.

Join a food co-op. Co-ops purchase food in bulk and often carry organic items. If there isn't one in your town, consider starting one with family and friends.

Share your knowledge. If you have discovered healthy organic or non-organic foods from a reputable supplier, pass the news on via an e-mail to MS organizations and friends. They will appreciate it immensely and you will help promote such suppliers, which eventually will be in a better position to lower prices based on demand.

Eating Out

Preferably, you should eat out no more than twice a week. Keep that time for the weekend with family and friends. Too many places use commercially packaged food and unhealthy fats, which are detrimental to your health. Not to mention how much salt is in those foods—and you might not get enough calcium either! It is extremely important that you pay attention to the type of foods you choose when going out.

In a restaurant, do not hesitate to question the waiter about the ingredients in a particular dish. Let him/her know you are on a specific diet and looking for high calcium dishes that are also low-fat. More and more chefs are willing to accommodate their clients today because they know it is important for the survival of the restaurant. There is also an increased demand for healthier choices, and the industry is paying attention. Choosing a restaurant that caters to foods closer to your diet is also wise—chances are you will find more food that you can enjoy there in the first place (e.g. Italian, Mediterranean, or vegetarian restaurants).

Quick Tips for Ordering at a Restaurant

- Order steamed vegetables with olive oil or lemon on the side
- Brown rice is also safe
- Ask for your dish to be prepared with a little olive oil, canola oil, or grapeseed oil, and no butter. Ask for olive oil and vinegar on the side for your salad dressing or bring your own dressing. Half a lemon is also a good substitute for dressing or butter on steamed vegetables.
- Half a baked potato is safe as long as it is without toppings and butter (you can always drizzle a little olive oil over it yourself).
- Stay away from unhealthy carbohydrates and ask to substitute steamed vegetables instead. Avoid most desserts except fresh fruits. It is best to save your sweet tooth for homemade, healthier goodies.
- Don't blindly eat what is served to you—pay attention to the type of food and the amount of food, and try to figure out the total calories. Put that into perspective with your meal allowance.

When visiting with family or friends, make them aware of your health situation a few days before the visit. If they already know, just give them a quick phone call to remind them, as many people have a very active lifestyle and may easily forget. Be very diligent and carefully choose what you eat. If needed, ask the host if he or she made the food from scratch, what is in it, or if it is store bought food. And remember: when in doubt, do not eat it. If you are not sure of the situation, you can always eat before you go to an event. If you know that the food the host will prepare will not agree with you, you can ask if you can bring your own food. No one should get upset; after all it is about making sure everyone enjoys the party!

While traveling, keep the same attitude that you have when you are eating out close to home. Be even more vigilant. It is best to bring your own food, but sometimes this is not possible (such as when traveling by airplane.) When booking your flight, most airlines will gladly reserve a low-fat meal for you. Vegetarian meals may be good, as they are often based on cheese and carbohydrates. Ask specifically what foods are included in the meals. At the airport, look for food that is freshly prepared in front of you and as close as possible to your nutritional plan. Take with you enough snack foods to last you a day or two in case of schedule delays. Nuts, raisins, and dates are easy to carry. You will be able to find bottles of water or milk in most places.

When traveling abroad, be even more careful than you would be at home. Foods are not prepared the same way and many unknown ingredients may be a real problem to your health. Stick with plain grilled, steamed, broiled, or baked main courses with rice, potatoes, or steamed vegetables as side dishes. If you have no choice, pick the healthiest option and eat what you know is safe for you. Be careful with raw foods, as sanitation may not be as thorough as at home. Always ask for a bottle of water to be opened in front of you. Don't miss the opportunity to go to a local market and purchase some fresh fruits, vegetables, and healthy snacks such as almonds, walnuts, hazelnuts, dates, or whatever you may be able to keep in your hotel room.

Don't forget to wash the vegetables and fruits with a bottle of water mixed with a little vinegar. This will help kill bacteria not visible to the eye. If you have a refrigerator in the room, stock it with milk, yogurt, or cheese to meet your daily calcium needs. Read all food labels carefully. If you don't understand the language, this may be a problem. See if the concierge or a person speaking your language at the hotel can assist you. Be on your guard at all times. If you take supplements or specific medications, make sure you have enough for your trip, plus a week's worth as back-up. Standards overseas are not always the same as in the United States.

Chapter 4

Foods to Avoid, Foods to Choose

Nutrition

To improve your health, you need to take care of yourself and the first step is to respect your body by giving it the food that will benefit it the most. Your meals should include a wide selection of fresh wholesome foods to satisfy not only your personal taste, but also your nutritional needs. Eating a variety of food is also important to avoid boredom and get the proper nutrients. As explained earlier, it is not always easy particularly during the winter when certain vegetables and fruits are not available or when you don't feel well. Substitution with organic frozen or canned foods is then necessary and only encouraged during such times.

You may also have to take into consideration your food sensitivities or allergies. At first, this can be difficult to deal with. Take time to think and be patient, soon you will realize it is not really a big deal and there are many ways to deal with it. If you think you may have allergies and have not yet been tested, be sure to contact your medical provider. This is very important as often foods can trigger aching pains, weakness, headaches, and many other symptoms.

When dealing with food sensitivities or allergies, think about how you can replace the offending food with something that you like and that has similar, if not healthier, nutritional values. For example, you can't eat cow milk, which is an important source of calcium that MS patients need, and you love cream of broccoli. Just substitute fortified unsweetened soy milk for cow milk in your favorite recipe—problem solved! Be aware, though, that soy milk does not offer the same nutrition value as cow milk. Look for a brand that has Vitamin A, Vitamin D, and Calcium added.

How much food should you eat? For sure, most of us have a natural desire to eat more than we really need. Knowing that, all we have to do is be sure to eat less and watch out for the food that our body does not really need or should not receive. It may be a simple formula, but it is very effective.

Which foods are most beneficial to a person with MS? As was said earlier, the secret lies in consuming a vast diversity of food that agrees with you, in the right quantities. Eating more foods containing anti-inflammatory properties is also beneficial. To select the right food for your body, you need to understand the basics about nutrients. Here is some very basic information to help you.

Carbohydrates are a main source of energy for the body (calories) and are necessary for the proper use of fats by the body. Complex carbohydrates are better for you and are found in many grains, dried beans, sweet potatoes, potatoes, corn, or cream of millet. Fibrous complex carbohydrates are found in broccoli, carrots, cauliflower, green beans, peppers, spinach, zucchini, and many other vegetables. Simple carbohydrates are found in many sugary items such as cereals, breakfast bars, crackers, candies, and many commercial desserts. Those are not healthy for you. On the other hand, simple carbohydrates found in small amounts in fruits such as apples, bananas grapefruit, oranges, pears, pineapples, or peaches are healthy for you and should be part of your daily allowances. Unrefined carbohydrates can possibly be a problem for some MS patients and are found in brown rice, wheat flour, and many products containing wheat. These can be important in a diet as they help eliminate waste and substitution needs to be explored carefully.

Fats are an indispensable part of every cell. They are a source of energy (calories), supply essential fatty acids and carry fat-soluble vitamins. Hormones are manufactured from fats, which make healthy fats indispensable to the good functioning of our body and even promote weight loss. Fats are also a good source of lubrication for the joints. There are three types of fats: saturated, polyunsaturated, and monounsaturated.

- *Saturated fats* are fats that raise bad cholesterol levels and are associated with heart disease. They are solid at room temperature and are found in animal products such as meat, poultry, eggs, dairy, packaged foods, and solid shortenings. The worst of these is hydrogenated fat (or partially hydrogenated), also called trans fat, which is found in many processed foods and should be eliminated from your diet. Check labels carefully. Coconut oil, palm oil, and non-dairy creamers contain high levels of saturated fats and should be eliminated as well.

- *Unsaturated fats (monounsaturated and polyunsaturated)* are healthier for you, but keep in mind that they are still fats, and that you should carefully control your daily intake. Monounsaturated fats have one double bond in their chemical structure and are liquid at room temperature. They lower bad cholesterol and raise levels of good cholesterol. They are found in olive oil, canola oil, or avocado oil.
- *Polyunsaturated fats* have two or more double bonds in their chemical structure and are liquid at room temperature. They have positive effects on blood sugar levels, reduce inflammation, and even influence the amount of fat stored by the body. They are found in fish oil, flaxseed oil, grapeseed oil, and walnut oil.

Proteins are a good source of energy and the major building materials for all body tissues. They also help produce enzymes and hormones, which regulate the body's functions. You'll find proteins in meats, poultry, fish, eggs, dairies, dried beans, legumes, soy (edamame), tofu, and nuts. Vegetable protein and lean animal protein (chicken, turkey, fish, egg whites, and low-fat dairies) are recommended. Eating proteins containing a large amount of healthy unsaturated fat, particularly Omega-3 fatty acids, is also essential for your well-being. Those can be found in fatty fish such as salmon, tuna, sardines, or anchovies.

Vitamins are chemical compounds found in many foods which help regulate the body's functions and fight infectious diseases. Contrary to belief, vitamins do not provide energy. Vitamins B (meats, poultry, nuts, legumes, green vegetables, dairies, and whole grains) and C (citrus, berries, green vegetables, papayas, tomatoes, livers, and potatoes) are not stored in the body and need to be eaten every day. However Vitamins A (dairies, green leafy vegetables, yellow vegetables, livers, and fruits), Vitamin D (dairy products, eggs, tuna, cod, mackerel, sea bass, liver oils, and sunlight), E (vegetable oils, dark green leafy vegetables, nuts, wheat germ, and whole grains) and K (dark green leafy vegetables, alfalfa, and tomatoes) are stored by the body.

Minerals are essential for the body to function properly and play an important role in our metabolic process. Minerals do not provide energy. Calcium (milk products, salmon, broccoli, and oysters), Chromium (onion, broccoli, meat, lettuce, and grape juice), Copper (vegetables, liver, legumes, cereals, and oil), Iodine (seafood, yeast breads, dairy products, eggs, and wheat germ), Iron (beef, poultry, beans, lentils, tofu, eggs, dark green leafy vegetables, broccoli, asparagus, grains, and dried fruits), Magnesium (dark green leafy vegetables, watercress, Brazil nuts, sunflower seeds, sesame seeds, pumpkin seeds, bananas, cashews, tofu, vegetables, and legumes), Manganese (grains, cereals, tea, pineapple, strawberries, and starches), Sodium (salt), Potassium (fruits, vegetables, meat, and milk), Selenium (meat, seafood, grains, molasses, and Brazil nuts), and Zinc (oyster, meat, dairy products, eggs, and wheat germ) are all minerals.

Fibers cannot be used by the body and therefore do not supply energy. However, they are important for the proper function of the intestines and may prevent cancers. Soluble fibers slow down the absorption of food in the stomach, and may be associated with reducing blood cholesterol, and maintaining the proper blood sugar level. Soluble fibers are found in oats, dried beans, lentils, peas, fruits, and vegetables. Insoluble fibers speed the digestive system and may reduce the risk of cancers. You find them in whole grains, dried beans, cereals, brown rice, and wheat pasta.

Water is indispensable for the body to function well. Water regulates the body temperature, assists in the digestive process, and transports nutrients and waste. Water is present in mostly everything, but certain foods contain much higher amounts of water than others (watermelon is mostly water). Drink plenty of water throughout the day. Water can also be used for making tea. The best known anti-inflammatory sources for tea are white and green tea. They also help stimulate the immune system and help to get rid of free radicals which are harmful to the body. Pure organic cranberry juice, no sugar added, is helpful with urinary tract infection, but should be drunk only when necessary, as it has a negative effect on bone density. Pure organic prune juice will also help with constipation.

Every nutrient's role is to supply energy to the body. That energy is measured in calories. Carbohydrates, proteins, and fats can be used by the body to supply energy.

- 1 gram of carbohydrate supplies 4 calories
- 1 gram of protein supplies 4 calories
- 1 gram of fat supplies 9 calories

As you can see, fats contribute a lot more calories which is why you need to keep your fat intake in line to stay healthy.

Now that you understand the role of nutrients, how many do you really need to function well? **For most people, the general healthy guideline is about 1400-1500 daily calories for women and 2000 to 2100 daily calories for men.** Keep in mind that those numbers may vary based on your lifestyle, level of activity and exercise, and if you are trying to gain or lose weight. Consult your physician or registered dietitian for your adequate daily calories.

To emphasize good healthy habits, we also need a healthy meal plan. Such a plan must emphasize a low-fat diet that contains healthy fats and high fiber intake. As a guideline, a meal should contain one portion of protein-rich foods (3 to 4 ounces for women and 6 to 7 ounces for men), one or more portions of vegetables low in starch (1 cup for women and 2 cups for men), and one portion of healthy whole grains or vegetables high in starch (1/2 cup for women and 3/4 cup for men of cooked whole grains or a small potato for women and a little larger for men). If weight loss is desired, limit your carbohydrates and starches (potatoes, rice, pasta, baked beans, yams, or sweet potatoes). This includes vegetables and fruits that contain high sugar levels (corn, peas, squash, plantains, or bananas). You should also eat two portions of fruits daily, preferably with breakfast, lunch, or a snack. On a daily basis, every meal should include an organic low-fat dairy product such as low-fat milk (cow or fortified soy milk), low-fat plain yogurt, and low-fat cheeses. Finally, drink plenty of water throughout the day to hydrate and to help cleanse the body of toxins.

Special Comments

Red meats are not prohibited but should be eaten occasionally. You may treat yourself every two weeks with 3 ounces of organic beef (for women) and 4 ounces of organic beef (for men). It is best to substitute beef with buffalo, venison, ostrich, or elk, which have less saturated fat. Buffalo and venison are very similar in taste to beef. Lamb, liver, kidney, heart, or tongue may also be eaten on rare occasion. Make sure the meat is always from an organic source.

Shellfish such as shrimp, crabs, lobsters, oysters, snails, mussels, clams, and scallops are not prohibited for those who have no cholesterol problems. They can be easily enjoyed once a week in soups, salads, or entrees.

Preferably organic canned or frozen foods are permissible when some seasonal products are not available or when you are not up to preparing fresh food. Organic is preferable. If purchasing non-organic, watch for hydrogenated fats or unhealthy fats, flours, sodium, thickeners, colorings, preservatives, additives, and any other ingredients that may cause you problems. Choose foods that are low in fat and prepared with olive oil or canola oil rather than other types of oils or butter.

Eliminate convenience foods, commercially prepared mixes, prepared packaged meals (including frozen ones) most foods from vending machines, baked goods containing refined white flour and unhealthy fats, most food bars, powders drinks, and commercial meal shakes. If you are not feeling well and cannot cook for yourself, see that your caregiver or helper does not feed you such foods, but rather prepares meals that are suitable for your needs and based on this book's recommendations. If neither of these possibilities are available to you, order fresh "home-style" meals from a couple of reliable sources. Establish a rapport with local places that offer healthy foods and that you can rely on with just a phone call. Your health is worth the time invested and, who knows, you may have fun doing it!

A word on eggs: Egg yolks contain cholesterol. If you have no problem with cholesterol, you may enjoy a whole egg. On the other hand, if you have to watch your cholesterol, use egg whites only. One whole egg equals two egg whites. Do not use commercial egg products as they may contain thickeners and can often cause allergic or sensitivity reactions.

A word on cooking chicken and turkey: Those white meats may be cooked once in awhile with the skin to preserve moisture, but do not eat the skin because it is high in fat.

A word on alcohol: Because this is a low-fat diet, digestion is much faster which causes alcohol to be absorbed faster through the bloodstream. Consequently, alcohol goes faster to the brain and people have reported lightheadedness, headache, hot sensations, a loss of mental capacities, stomach and body cramps, fatigue, confusion, or even feeling drunk and hung over after just a small amount of alcohol. Many mixed drinks and commercial mixes contain ingredients that can cause health problems. So it is best to totally stay away from alcohol.

A healthy tip on constipation: You can take 1 teaspoon to 2 teaspoons maximum of cod fish oil or flaxseed oil daily. Or you can also have up to 1 tablespoon freshly ground flaxseeds daily mixed in your food. A few prunes, pre-soaked in water for 24 hours, after a meal will also be helpful. When traveling, use pills for convenience but do so for short-term periods only. Individual flaxseed sachets might be available at your local health food stores.

Hydration and fiber also play an important role in preventing constipation. Drink lots of water throughout the day and add fiber to your meals (vegetables and fruits). Natural organic prune juice, no sugar added, is also very helpful with constipation.

Chapter 5

Tips on Shopping

Selecting Food

As we just explained, nutrition is very important and so is the food we choose. You need to be concerned with colors, shapes, flavors, textures, personal likes and dislikes, allergies and sensitivities, diet, and foods that complement each other. These factors are all important in helping to avoid sickness, boredom, and unpleasant experiences.

Colors and shapes give a dish an attractive appearance and are pleasing to the eyes. Flavors and textures excite our taste buds, which send signals to our brain and, in turn, send us back sensations. Those sensations can be good or bad. They can come to you within seconds, minutes, hours, or even over-night. During that time allergies, food sensitivities, or food poisoning can occur. Flavors need to be in harmony, not over powering, not too light. For example, acidic and tart foods as accompaniments to fatty foods help balance the taste and promote easier digestion.

Softness and firmness is what is referred to as **texture.** Vegetables taste much better when crunchy rather than mushy, and don't forget they retain more vitamins and minerals when they are not overcooked. Creating a meal with similar textures is boring and not recommended (eg. leek and potato soup, mashed potato, and meatloaf).

Personal preference is another important point because none of us will eat something we don't like. How your body responds to what you eat is equally important. No one wants to eat something that makes you sick. Likes and dislikes are important to consider when selecting foods as long as you don't forget that nutrients are even more important to your well-being. You might have to tolerate foods you dislike once in awhile for your health's sake. Find ways with herbs, spices, or sauces to camouflage the flavors of healthy foods that you don't particularly like. In other words, trick your taste buds! Here is a quick trick to deal with strong flavors that may bother you. Take, for example, cauliflower. Once cooked, cauliflower can have strong flavors that turn people off. To avoid such a problem, all you need to do is to cook the cauliflower in milk. The strong flavors will be absorbed by the milk and the cauliflower will taste milder and even sweeter. If smell is still a problem, mix the cauliflower with another ingredient such as mashed potatoes with garlic and herbs. The cauliflower flavor will disappear, but not the nutrients! If you think that way about food, you will enjoy your food much more and will have fun creating your own recipe while still enjoying all the benefits of such healthy foods. Be careful to choose combinations that make sense. In this case, it would not be advisable to experiment mixing cauliflower with mint—they don't complement each other, and taste quite awful together! As you can see, all these factors are important in selecting the right food.

Reading Labels

Strive to purchase fresh ingredients and prepare the food yourself. But from time to time, you may have to purchase organic prepared, canned, or frozen foods. If so, you must read the entire label carefully. Most packaged foods will offer important nutritional information. A label will offer nutrition facts which will be broken down into serving size, number of servings, amount per serving, calories, total fat, cholesterol, trans-fat, carbohydrates, protein, sodium, sugar, and vitamins. Be particularly aware of the fats, sodium, carbohydrates, and calcium. Vitamin D is often not shown.

For carbohydrates, you will often see two categories: fiber and sugar. Remember that sugar can come from many sources. The label should specify the origin (such as sugar, brown sugar, turbinado sugar, honey, maple sugar or syrup, sucrose, glucose, corn syrup, dextrin, confectioner's sugar, high fructose, lactose, dextrose, maltodextrin, molasses, caramel, date sugar, rice syrup, etc.) Sugar can also come from sugar alcohol: sorbitol, xylitol, lactitol, isomalt, maltitol, or mannitol. These sugars have fewer total calories than regular sugar. You will find them often in low-calorie, low-carb, reduced-carb, and even carb-free products. However, they have been found to cause various negative reactions such as nausea, headaches, diarrhea, bloating, and even allergies. You should try to stay away from those products whenever possible. Avoid aspartame and any products containing aspartame as it may cause cancer.

Be aware that manufacturers do not always report the exact numbers because they are allowed to round numbers down. If the number is less than 0.5 g, they don't have to report it either. So carefully read the list of ingredients to look for unhealthy fats, bad sugars, and other ingredients that may cause health problems.

Familiarize yourself as much as possible with labels and read carefully every time you buy a product. When shopping, take with you the list of foods and ingredients you cannot eat. When in doubt about an ingredient, do not purchase the product. Always compare nutritional ingredients among products until you are familiar with them. Once you find a brand that agrees with you, don't ever assume it will be around forever. Manufacturers are known to change a few ingredients now and then for various reasons. For example, they may find an ingredient from a cheaper source overseas. So read the label every time you purchase a product.

Here is a label example (walnut pieces):

Nutrition Facts

Serving Size 1 oz (30g)
Serving Per Container 15 Servings

Amount Per Serving

Calories 210   Calories from fat 180

	% Daily Value*
Total Fat 20g	31%
Saturated Fat 1.5g	8%
Trans Fat 0g	
Cholesterol 0mg	0%
Sodium 0mg	
Total Carbohydrates 3g	
Dietary Fiber 3g	14%
Sugar 0g	
Protein 5g	

Vitamin A 0%	Vitamin C 0%
Calcium 2%	Iron 6%

There are 9 calories/gram of fat. Since there are 20g of fat in this product, 180 of the total calories (9X20=180) are from fat.

5% Daily Value or less is low – 20% Daily Value or more is high

Actual grams of fat in this product

It is mandatory that trans fat be listed on labels since 2006

Actual amount of cholesterol in this product

Actual amount of sodium in this product

Total of carbohydrates from various sources

Dietary fiber from the total amount of carbohydrates

Total sugar in the amount of carbohydrates listed

Total protein in this product

Shopping List

Below are three lists that can be used for MS patients' diet guidelines. You will find **"Encouraged Foods," "Questionable Foods, no more than once a week,"** and **"Prohibited Foods."** Keep in mind that everyone's metabolism is different and no one list fits all. Where one person may find relief in not eating a particular food, another person may not. Consequently, it is very important to start to work on your own personal list. The lists below are a good start to help you design your own healthy diet. A personal diet needs to be carefully designed for each individual and possibly include "vitamin and mineral" supplementation to compensate for loss of natural sources (please consult your physician). Keeping a journal is highly recommended, as it may help you determine reasons for when you are not feeling well or when you are feeling great.

Once you have established your own list of foods to avoid, you will be able to make substitutions for your recipes and enjoy your meals without any worries. Finding a balanced diet and lifestyle that makes you feel great will also make a difference in your overall sense of well-being, and you must maintain your new diet and lifestyle for the rest of your life. If you do so, your overall well-being will be enhanced permanently and, consequently, you will be able to live a more pleasurable life. Patience, perseverance, discipline, self-esteem, self-confidence, faith, engaging in relaxation techniques, and eating right are all habits that will contribute to your well-being.

	Safe and Encouraged Foods	Questionable Foods Permissible	Prohibited Foods
Cereals/Flour/ starch	Millet, buckwheat, quinoa, amaranth, oats, nut flours, wild rice, wheat germ, brown rice, whole wheat pasta, chestnuts, potato, sweet potato, tapioca, whole wheat couscous	Corn, oats, muesli, nut flours, barley, rye, spelt, bulgur, semolina, wheat germ, wheat or products containing gluten due to possible allergies. Careful with brown rice, whole wheat pasta, and yeast due to possible allergies or sensitivities	Chips, crackers, many cereals, commercial breads made with refined flour, refined grains, white rice and regular pasta
Fats	Preference to: Olive oil, canola oil, grapeseed oil, avocado oil, flaxseed oil, fish oil, and walnut oil.	Nut oils due to possible allergies.	Limit the use of corn oil, peanut oil, sesame oil, soybean oil, sunflower oil, safflower oil

	Safe and Encouraged Foods	Questionable Foods Permissible	Prohibited Foods
Meat, Fish, and Eggs	White meat from turkey and chicken. Fish: wild salmon, tuna, sardines, herring, anchovies, cod, mackerel, halibut, snapper, founder, sole, shark, mahi mahi, perch, and most lean white fish. Can salmon or tuna in water. Can sardines in olive oil or tomato sauce. Organic eggs.	Cornish hen, pheasant, and rabbit. Eggs may cause allergy reaction.	No dark meat (chicken and turkey). Avoid red meats the first year (beef, buffalo, venison). No lamb, mutton, pork, goose, duck, sausages, patés, or bacon. No liver, kidney, heart, and tongue. No commercial lunch meat. No eggs substitutes
Vegetables, Legumes, and Fruits	All and particularly: carrots, squash, beets, zucchinis, broccolis, potatoes, sweet potatoes, onions, garlic, leeks, turnips, chestnuts, peas, yams, garbanzos, cabbages, pumpkins, green leafy vegetables, bell peppers, beans, lentils, cauliflower, tomatoes, avocadoes, ginger, apples, pears, grapes, pineapple, mangos, cantaloupes, papayas, apricots, peaches, citrus, grapes, berries, kiwis, unsweetened dried fruits (without sulfite and preservatives)	Allergies or sensitivities are always possible with any of those listed vegetables and fruits. Most often reported are: green beans, spinach, bell peppers, onions, garlic, tomatoes, strawberries, or citrus Fried or commercially breaded or coated with a batter vegetables, vegetables cooked in butter, vegetables bouillons or cubes, prepared vegetables containing thickeners, high fat, and high sodium.	Sweetened and flour-coated dried fruits
Dairies	Low fat dairies (milk, buttermilk, sour cream, plain yogurt, plain yogurt with added fresh fruits, cottage cheese, cheese, rice milk, soy milk, almond milk, hazelnut milk	Homemade custards and puddings, spreadable low fat cheese, milk based beverages, or rice dream products. Homemade low fat frozen yogurt or ice cream. Rice milk, soy milk, or almond or hazelnut milk due to possible allergies.	Full fat dairies and desserts (milk, cream, butter, margarine, sour cream, whipped cream, cheese, yogurt, ice cream, cottage cheese, imitation dairies, custards, puddings, and products containing unhealthy fats.

	Safe and Encouraged Foods	Questionable Foods Permissible	Prohibited Foods
Condiments	Apple cider vinegar, herbs, spices, salts, peppers, mustards, ketchup, hot sauce, homemade low fat dressing	Balsamic vinegar, wine vinegar, ketchup, barbecue sauce, herbs, spices, hot sauce. Careful with spices mix as they may contain other ingredients.	Broth cubes or dry mixes, most commercial prepared sauces, commercial dressings
Desserts, Sweets, And Nuts	Maple syrup, honey, agave nectar, fruit fructose, preserves Raw almonds, walnuts, hazelnuts, pistachios, pumpkin seeds, pepitas and flaxseeds	Fructose, dextrose, brown sugar, agar agar, marmalades, jams, homemade low fat desserts, low fat rice or tapioca puddings Peanut, sesame seeds	Corn syrup, Stevia, NutraSweet, Splenda, Saccharine, Aspartame, and any artificial sweeteners. Gelatin, all packaged commercial mixes or desserts, commercial baked goods, chewing gums, high fat desserts Sweetened and coated dried fruits
Beverages and Extracts	Water (tap, sparkling, or bottled), white tea, green tea, black tea, or herbal teas. Homemade fruit juice, homemade concentrated fruit juices, organic prunes juice (no sugar added)	Regular or decaffeinated coffee, white, green, and black teas, Organic natural unsweetened commercial fruit juices	Sodas, high caffeine drinks, some carbonated drinks, flavored waters, powdered base mixes for drinks or shakes, artificial flavored or colored drinks, coffee substitute, artificial syrups, sweetened fruit juices. Chocolate and cacao. No vanilla extracts which often contains alcohol. Alcohol beverages

Chapter 6

Prepping Your Kitchen

Cooking with the Right Tools

Because you may find yourself tired, it is important for you to limit energy expenditure in the kitchen. There is no better way to do this than having the right tools to help you out. Having a food processor, electric mixer, blender, microwave, good quality knives, electric can opener, and utensils within easy reach while prepping and cooking will contribute to making your life easier. Other important tools in your kitchen are your pots and pans. A good quality pan distributes heat evenly over the entire surface and allows proper cooking. Though a heavy-gauge pan is better for cooking, it may be a problem to lift for some patients. When looking for lighter pans, it is important that the weight of the metal be on the bottom of the pan. This allows for better conductivity and consequently better, faster cooking. Different kinds of metals are available and you should be concerned with the conductivity of heat rather than appearance.

- **Copper** is the best heat conductor, but rather expensive. Copper reacts chemically with some foods, which can have poisonous results. Lining it with another metal, such as stainless steel, avoids such problems.
- **Aluminum** is a very good conductor and commonly used. Do not use aluminum cookware for storing strong acidic foods, since it will chemically react with the food, creating poisonous compounds.
- **Calphalon**, which is made of anodized aluminum, is a better choice if you are concerned about any chemical reactions.
- **Stainless steel** is a poor heat conductor and, therefore, not recommended.

- **Cast iron** is a great conductor but can be very heavy. It holds heat for a long time, but has the disadvantage of cracking easily when hit or dropped. When you scratch and wash your pan, then dry it, you will notice a black stain on your cloth. This means that a small amount of iron can leak into your food presenting a health concern. Avoid using such pans.
- **Non-stick** such as Teflon is ideal for low-fat cooking. Make sure the surface is always perfect. One little dent will allow the metal under the Teflon layer to come into contact with the food. This can be a serious health issue. Inspect regularly and replace immediately any pans that have even the smallest scratch.
- **Earthenware** and glass are easily breakable. They are not good conductors, but resist corrosion and do not have chemical reactions with acidic foods like some metal pans do. These are good for baking casseroles, though.

Seasoning, Herbs, and Spices

You may wonder what the difference is between seasonings and flavoring, and why this is important. It is important, particularly with low-fat cooking. Since fat provides flavor and you are going to limit fat in your cooking, you need to find other ways to compensate for it and enhance your cuisine. There is no better way than by using seasonings, herbs, and spices.

Seasoning means enhancing and balancing the natural flavors of a dish by adding salt and pepper. You will notice that the recipes in this book use a very little amount of salt. The reason is that our foods are too salty these days, and you actually need very little to balance flavors and for your health. Various types of salt are available: table salt, granulated salt, coarse salt, sea salt, and mineral salt. I prefer sea salt because it is un-processed and contains important minerals and trace elements. It also gives a much better flavor to food in very small quantities. Peppers are available in many different forms: black, white, green, red, etc. It is best to freshly grind pepper to obtain a dish's full flavor.

Flavoring means adding one or more flavors to a dish without overpowering the original flavor (unless purposely done). Flavoring refers to anything other than salt and pepper, for example: lemon juice, herbs, spices, vegetables, mustard, lemon or orange peel, red or cayenne pepper (no, they do not belong to the pepper family but rather the paprika and sweet bell pepper family), low-sodium soy sauce, etc.

Herbs are the leaves of plants and spices are the buds, fruits, flowers, seeds, roots of plants and trees. Keep dried herbs and spices in a cool place, away from lights and heat (not next to the stovetop or oven) or they will spoil quickly. Keep them tightly covered. Most of the dry herbs have a shelf life of four to six months. Do not buy large quantities since you probably will not use them.

Also, buy high quality herbs—if you buy poor quality, you end up putting more in your food, and thus spending more money.

Fresh herbs with short stems should be stored in an unsealed plastic bag or wrapped in a moist paper towel. Always refrigerate herbs so they can keep up to a week. Fresh herbs with long stems should be placed in the refrigerator

Below is a list of herbs and spices that go best with certain foods.

Use a few per dish, not all. Explore them, use them, and then be adventurous and create your own combination. This is what will make you familiar with them and make your cooking experience most exciting.

Chicken
Chervil, coriander, cumin, marjoram, parsley, peppers, rosemary, sage, savory, shallot, basil, tarragon, thyme, and ginger

Beef, Buffalo, or Venison
Dill, leek, marjoram, oregano, parsley, peppers, rosemary, savory, basil, tarragon, thyme, ginger, garlic, and shallot

Veal
Leek, marjoram, oregano, parsley, peppers, rosemary, savory, basil, tarragon, thyme, ginger, garlic, and shallot

Rabbit
Oregano, parsley, peppers, rosemary, thyme, ginger, garlic, and shallot

Seafood
Anise, dill, marjoram, oregano, parsley, peppers, rosemary, sage, basil, tarragon, thyme, ginger, garlic, and shallot

Fruit
Ambrosia, anise, mint, parsley, rosemary, sage, sesame, and ginger

Vegetables
Chives, cumin, dill, leek, marjoram, mint, oregano, parsley, peppers, paprika, rosemary, sage, basil, tarragon, thyme, ginger, garlic, and shallot

Salads
Ambrosia, anise, caraway, chervil, chives, dandelion, fennel, leek, mint, garlic, mustard, oregano, parsley, peppers, rosemary, savory, shallot, basil, tarragon, and ginger

Eggs
Chives, cumin, leek, marjoram, oregano, parsley, peppers, tarragon, paprika, and shallot

Pickles
Coriander, mint, peppers, savory, shallot, and ginger

in an open plastic bag or at room temperature (if cool) in a small amount of water. It is best to find fresh herbs with their roots still intact since they will keep fresh and flavorful longer. Wrap the roots in a damp paper towel and cover with a plastic bag. Refrigerate, leaving the leaves out in the open. They can keep up to a week.

If you grow your own herbs, the best time to pick them is in the morning after the dew has evaporated. Do not wash until use. When using fresh herbs remember that they lose their flavor very quickly, so use them towards the end of cooking. Use dry herbs for long cooking and finish with fresh herbs for added flavor.

Using herbs and spices as an enhancement to a dish is one of the most important parts of great healthy cooking. But use them carefully. It is always easy to add but impossible to remove. Remember that you may have possible sensitivities or allergies to some herbs and spices. So be careful and keep notes in your journal and cooking recipes book.

Finally, here are examples of various herbs mixes that you can create at home.

Creole: 2 tsp. salt, 2 ½ Tbsp. paprika, 2 Tbsp. garlic powder, 1 Tbsp. dry oregano, 1 Tbsp. black pepper, 1 Tbsp. cayenne pepper, 1 Tbsp. onion powder, 1 Tbsp. dry thyme

Italian: 1 Tbsp. dry basil, 1/4 tsp. dry rosemary, ¼ tsp. dry thyme, ¼ tsp. dry marjoram, ¼ tsp. dry oregano, 1 Tbsp. dry parsley

Bouquet garni: 1 bay leaf, 3 sprigs fresh thyme, 4 sprigs fresh parsley, 1 garlic clove, 2 celery stalks, 2 pieces leek (green part only), 10 peppercorns

Fine herbs or salad herbs: 1 tsp. fresh chervil, 1 tsp. fresh chives, 1 tsp. fresh tarragon, 1 tsp. fresh parsley

Persillade: 2 large garlic cloves, ½ cup parsley, 3 Tbsp. shallots

Provence herbs: 1 Tbsp. dry thyme, 1 Tbsp. dry savory, 1 Tbsp. marjoram, 1 Tbsp. dry basil, 1 tsp. dry fennel, 1 Tbsp. dry rosemary, 2 dry bay leaf crumbled

Asian: 1 Tbsp. garlic powder, 1 Tbsp. ground ginger, 1/2 tsp. ground cumin, 1 tsp. coriander, 1 tsp. curry powder, ½ tsp. cayenne pepper, ½ tsp. dry mustard, 1/4 tsp. celery seeds, 1/4 tsp. nutmeg.

Part III

The Meals

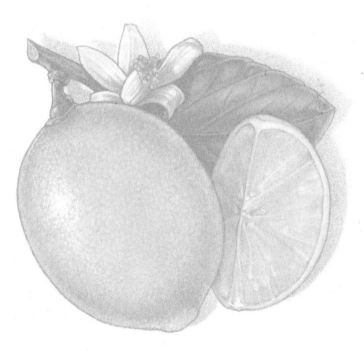

Chapter 7

A Chef's Secrets for Easy, Quick Meals

Healthy Cooking Methods

Multiple Sclerosis patients must **pay particular attention to the amount of fat used in cooking.** The use of Teflon pans helps in such cases. Limit the use of olive oil, canola oil, or grapeseed oil to a minimum. It is already done for you in these recipes. Use steaming, baking, grilling, broiling, or par-boiling methods as often as possible. For stir-fried and sautéing methods, using Teflon and very little oil is recommended. Brush the oil on the bottom of the pan or spray from your own pump spray bottle. Stay away from commercial oil spray that may contain fillers and other unhealthy ingredients. To thicken sauces, substitute arrowroot or cornstarch to the often found flour or beurre manié in recipes. There is no exact amount of thickening agent to give you, as the amount of arrowroot/cornstarch and water mixture may vary depending on the amount of water rendered by the ingredients involved or the reduction process. In these recipes, you will see cornstarch, but you can substitute arrowroot in the same way. A little secret to obtaining the right thickness for a sauce is to dip a spoon in the sauce, turn it over, and make a line across with your finger. Tilt over the spoon. If the sauce does not run over the line, it is the perfect thickness. If it does, you need to thicken with a little cornstarch-water mixture. Start with a spoon and see how it reacts after boiling. If it gets too thick, just add a little liquid to thin out.

Cooking Vegetables

When cooking vegetables, follow those basic directions:
- **For white vegetables** (onion, cauliflower, white cabbage, celery, cucumber, zucchini, etc.), use a little lemon juice or cream of tartar in the water to keep

them white. Do not use salt; they will turn yellowish.

- **For red vegetables** (example red cabbage), use an acid (vinegar) or cream of tartar to emphasize their red colors. Do not use salt; they will turn blue or blue-green.
- **For green vegetables** (broccoli, asparagus, green beans, etc.), use salt to emphasize a darker green color. Do not use acids or cream of tartar; they will turn olive green.
- **For yellow and orange vegetables or roots** (carrots, winter squash, sweet potatoes, tomatoes, red peppers, etc.), the use of acids or salt is not a problem.

Steam a variety of vegetables in one session. Once barely cooked, transfer them to an ice cold water bath to stop the cooking process. Pat dry and store separately in bags and place in the refrigerator. In a flash, you will be able to accompany a variety of dishes or snack on healthy foods. For a gourmet touch, drizzle a little bit of a prepared sauce (with your fish or chicken) over the vegetables and serve immediately. Remember lemon juice goes a long way and has no calories. Homemade tomato sauce is also a healthy choice, as it has the advantages of being low-fat and loaded with vitamins.

Remember, you do not have to eat only steamed or blanched vegetables to stay healthy. You can stir-fry them or sauté them with a little oil (1 teaspoon) once in awhile and use different flavorings. The key is to avoid boredom and keep eating those vegetables. Blanched vegetables can be stored in the refrigerator 5 days without affecting them, and no longer than 7 days.

There are many ways to prepare and enjoy vegetables and there is no need to be concerned with loss of vitamins, as long as you do not overcook your vegetables. Keep them al dente and you will do a big favor to your body.

Some Tips for Saving Time

- Double the amount of food you prepare in one cooking session. Example: buy a couple of whole chickens and roast them in the oven while you are doing something else. Then divide them up for three different meals. For each meal, serve them with a different sauce and steamed, roasted, or stir-fried vegetables. Freeze or refrigerate in appropriate storage containers.
- Cook several skinless chicken breasts on an oiled baking sheet. Brush a little flavored oil and season to taste. Cook under the broiler until golden brown, turn over and brush with more flavored oil. Finish cooking until cooked through. The whole cooking process may take you 20 to 30 minutes depending upon the thickness of the breasts. Let cool, package individually, and store appropriately for later use.

- Do the same with fish fillets or steaks. The cooking process is much faster, so watch out. It will take a maximum 10 to 15 minutes. If the fillets have a skin on one side, place the skin side down on the baking sheet.

- Serve each meal with a different sauce, lemon or lime wedges, and steamed, roasted, or stir-fried vegetables (see below for suggestions). Freeze or refrigerate in appropriate storage containers.

- Wash and dry various greens. Store in plastic containers or bags for quick salads. Lettuces don't freeze well, so only prepare what you will eat within three or four days. It is ok to purchase pre-packaged and pre-cut organic mixed vegetables when time is of the essence during physically challenged days. Make sure you wash them before use.

- Make a week's worth of salad dressing and store in the refrigerator. Here is a recipe:

  ### Ingredients:
  1 tablespoon Dijon Mustard
  1 cup olive oil
  ½ cup walnut oil
  ½ cup wine vinegar
  1 shallot, minced
  2 garlic cloves, minced
  4 tablespoons freshly minced salad herbs
  Salt and pepper to taste

  ### Directions:
  Place all the ingredients in a tall container and season to taste. With a hand blender, mix well. Add a little water to thin out, if desired. Refrigerate for up to a week.

- Pre-cut large amount of vegetables and fruits. Store them in plastic containers or bags for quick snacks and side dishes. They can also be stored cooked (blanched or steamed and placed in ice cold water to stop the cooking, then pat dry before storing) in the refrigerator or freezer. Make sure you pack each vegetable separately to avoid the transfer of odors to other vegetables. Date before freezing. When things are tough, you may consider purchasing organic pre-cut vegetables to make it easier on you. Make sure you wash them before use to avoid possible illness and any preservatives that still may be on them to allow for longer storage.

- Shred low-fat cheese and store in plastic bags. This is also cheaper than buying cheese already shredded. Cheese does not freeze well. Remember a little freshly shredded Parmesan sprinkled at the last minute over a dish can do the trick without adding too much fat.

- Double recipes to start to build inventory in the freezer for days you are tired or last minute emergencies. Stock the freezer with freshly cooked vegetables, homemade soups, stews, purées, rice, etc.
- Prepare some healthy instant snacks and store individual portions for quick use.
- Make your own broth/stock and store in ice cube trays or small plastic bags for individual portions and in larger bags for bigger portions. When purchasing commercial broth/stock look for organic products that are low-sodium, and low-fat. If not organic, make sure they are free-range (for chicken), free of preservatives, gluten, additives, or artificial colorings.
- Finally, do not hesitate to recruit helpers for a cooking session together. This is a great deal of fun. Choose a day you feel well and people are available to come to your home. Together, you can prepare a couple of weeks worth of meals while enjoying each other's company. Children should also be involved, as it is good to spend the time together and you can teach them about responsibilities and living a healthy lifestyle. They will also learn about sharing, working with others, and helping others. One warning: Be very careful not to get hurt, as a crowded, busy kitchen may become a hazardous situation for you.

Chapter 8

The Recipes

About the Recipes

Due to their illness, many Multiple Sclerosis patients lose interest in food, which really adversely affects their health and increases the chance of relapses. Consequently, **it is important to instill a passion for healthy and delicious food**s to awaken important senses and encourage MS patients to follow a healthier diet. Doing so will also contribute to a sense of responsibility towards personal health and overall better well-being. The healthy recipes selected for this book may be quite a change for you. Note, however, that there is nothing wrong with treating yourself with something less healthy once in a while. You can even do this once a week, as long as you stay within your recommended daily calories. Giving yourself occasional treat days will make it a lot easier to maintain a healthier diet overall and treating yourself is a must if you are to stay committed to your health and your happiness. Consider making small sacrifices by eating foods you don't particularly care for, that you know agree with you, for the sake of your health. Eventually, you will get used to these foods. After all, a healthy diet is about balance.

Many of these recipes include fresh ingredients. Occasionally commercial products may be called for, but try to keep these to a minimum and purchase organic products instead. Though some of the recipes might appear challenging, they are all really simple. Once you practice the healthy cooking techniques a few times, they will become easy. Don't let anyone discourage you in your attempt to learn new healthy cooking techniques and eat right. Perhaps they don't cook, don't know how, find cooking a waste of time, or not worth the effort. Show them how easy it is and how pleasurable it is to prepare and eat natural, healthy foods.

Finally, **do not be afraid to substitute ingredients in these recipes** to meet your personal needs. Recipes are meant to be changed. In fact, always consider a recipe book as a base or guideline for you, the cook. Bringing your own touch, knowing what you or your family likes, is what will make regular meals become extraordinary meals. So if you do not like Ahi, feel free to substitute another fish which has similar nutrients and that agrees with you. If you don't like the herbs, consult the list for guidelines and substitute herbs that you know you will enjoy. Be adventurous and experience the joy of cooking and eating healthy foods.

Breakfast

With the hectic pace of life today, spending a few minutes sitting down to eat breakfast seems the least of many people's concerns. This is a huge mistake. If you don't take the time to eat first thing in the morning, you will throw off your eating regimen for the rest of the day. **You don't have to indulge in a huge breakfast to give your body what it needs to get moving.** Organic cereals listed in the recipes are a quick and easy way to start your day, and they will give you a start on your needed calcium intake. When you have energy, enjoy a more complex breakfast recipe such as cheese blintzes. When preparing eggs, purchase organic or free-range eggs with Omega-3 fatty acids, which will provide you with healthier and more anti-inflammatory sources than regular eggs. Don't forget to hydrate with water, freshly squeezed juice, a homemade smoothie, or tea.

The following recipes are designed to jump-start your day and provide you with the physical and mental energy you will need to get through the morning. Over time you will notice that the first part of your day is a lot easier to handle when you provide your body with the nutrients it needs. Your energy boost is sure to increase your productivity—and encourage your metabolism to function better.

All-Bran with Apples and Cinnamon

serves 1

✓ *You may substitute low-fat milk with low-fat soy milk, low-fat rice milk, or low–fat almond milk.*

ingredients

1 cup all bran flakes
1/2 cup low-fat milk
1/4 cup apples
1 tablespoon raisins
1 teaspoon freshly ground flaxseeds
Cinnamon to taste (optional)

cooking instructions

In a bowl mix the cereal with the milk.
Top with the apples, raisins, and flaxseeds.
Sprinkle with cinnamon
and serve immediately.

nutritional facts

Per Serving (with 2% milk): 252 Cal (14% from Fat, 13% from Protein, 73% from Carb); 9 g Protein; 5 g Tot Fat; 2 g Sat Fat; 1 g Mono Fat; 52 g Carb; 9 g Fiber; 23 g Sugar; 192 mg Calcium; 12 mg Iron; 345 mg Sodium; 10 mg Cholesterol

Cream of Millet

serves 1

✔ *You may substitute low-fat almond milk with low-fat rice milk, low-fat soy milk, or low-fat milk and flaxseed oil with ground flaxseeds (up to 1 tablespoon). Feel free to exchange the peach for apricot, apple, mango, or berries.*

ingredients

1/4 cup pearl millet
3/4 cup to 1cup low-fat almond milk
1 teaspoon pumpkin pie spices
(optional)
1/2 peach, peeled and diced
2 teaspoons maple syrup
2 teaspoons slivered almonds
1 teaspoon flaxseed oil
Small pinch of salt

cooking instructions

Warm the 1 cup of milk, salt, and the spices over medium heat. Wash the millet a couple of times and drain well. Place the millet in a pan. Add the almonds and the warm flavored milk. Reduce heat and simmer for 20 minutes or until the liquid is absorbed.

Transfer to a serving bowl and mix in the maple syrup. Top with the fruits, drizzle with flaxseed oil, and serve immediately. When using less cooking liquid, the grain is fluffier and crunchier. Using more liquid will create a more moist, soft texture. This is about personal preferences, so experiment and find the texture you like.

nutritional facts

Per Serving: 384 Cal (19% from Fat, 15% from Protein, 65% from Carb); 15 g Protein; 8 g Tot Fat; 1 g Sat Fat; 2 g Mono Fat; 63 g Carb; 5 g Fiber; 25 g Sugar; 525 mg Calcium; 2 mg Iron; 132 mg Sodium; 5 mg Cholesterol

Homemade Granola

serves 10

ingredients

1/4 cup honey

1/4 cup grapeseed oil

2 teaspoons cinnamon

1 teaspoon almond extract

1 teaspoon orange extract

3 ½ cups rolled oats

1/4 cup slivered almonds

1/4 cup chopped walnuts

cooking instructions

Preheat the oven to 350°F. In a bowl, mix the honey, spices, oil, and extracts. Stir in the oats and nuts. Mix well and spread over a greased cookie sheet. Bake for 10 minutes. Stir and continue to bake for another 10 minutes, or until golden brown. Cool completely and break apart. Store in an airtight container away from heat.

You may substitute the honey with agave nectar. Enjoy with low-fat soy milk, low-fat rice milk, low-fat almond milk, low-fat milk, low-fat plain yogurt, or a mix of low-fat milk and low-fat plain yogurt. Top with your favorite fruits for added nutritional values.

Add 1 teaspoon freshly ground flaxseeds per serving before serving.

nutritional facts

Per Serving (1/2 cup granola):
231 Cal (41% from Fat, 9% from Protein, 50% from Carb); 6 g Protein;
11 g Tot Fat; 1 g Sat Fat;
3 g Mono Fat; 29 g Carb; 3 g Fiber;
10 g Sugar; 30 mg Calcium;
1 mg Iron; 2 mg Sodium;
0 mg Cholesterol

Oatmeal with Kiwi and Banana

serves 1

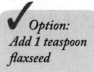

✓ *Option:
Add 1 teaspoon
flaxseed*

ingredients

1/2 cup to 3/4 cup oatmeal
1 cup to 1½ cup low-fat milk, hot
1 teaspoon almonds
1 kiwi, diced
1/2 banana, diced

cooking instructions

Mix the oatmeal with the hot milk until the liquid is incorporated. Add in the almonds, kiwi, banana, and serve immediately.

nutritional facts

Per Serving: 389 Cal (16% from Fat, 14% from Protein, 69% from Carb); 15 g Protein; 8 g Tot Fat; 3 g Sat Fat; 2 g Mono Fat; 72 g Carb; 10 g Fiber; 30 g Sugar; 339 mg Calcium; 2 mg Iron; 105 mg Sodium; 20 mg Cholesterol

Muesli with Berries

serves 1

ingredients

1/2 cup muesli cereal
1/2 cup low-fat plain yogurt
2 teaspoons almonds
2 ounces berries (about 2/5 cup)
Low-fat milk (to thin out, if desired)

cooking instructions

In a bowl, mix the cereal with the yogurt. If desired, thin out with a little milk. Top with the berries, raisins, and serve immediately.

nutritional facts

Per Serving: 277 Cal (20% from Fat, 16% from Protein, 64% from Carb); 12 g Protein; 7 g Tot Fat; 2 g Sat Fat; 3 g Mono Fat; 46 g Carb; 7 g Fiber; 24 g Sugar; 272 mg Calcium; 4 mg Iron; 214 mg Sodium; 7 mg Cholesterol

Sweet Potatoes and Buckwheat Pancakes

serves 3

✓ *You may substitute low-fat milk with low-fat soy milk, low-fat rice milk, or low-fat almond milk.*

ingredients

8 ounces sweet potatoes
(about 2 medium sweet potatoes)
3/4 cup buckwheat flour
1 tablespoon ground flaxseeds
1 egg or 2 egg whites
1/4 teaspoon salt
1/4 cup water
1/2 teaspoon cinnamon

1 ¼ cup low-fat milk
3 tablespoons maple syrup
2 tablespoons walnuts

cooking instructions

Cook the sweet potatoes in boiling water until a knife can easily be inserted in the potatoes, about 20 to 30 minutes.

Mix the flour, eggs, salt, water, cinnamon, and a little milk in a large bowl. Continue to add the milk until you obtain a smooth batter. Mash the sweet potatoes and mix in the prepared batter.

Heat a little canola oil in a large nonstick pan over medium heat. Using a ladle, pour enough batter to form 3 pancakes in the pan. Let the dough set and brown. Turn over with a spatula and cook until slightly browned. Serve immediately with maple syrup and walnuts.

nutritional facts

Per Serving (1 egg white): 364 Cal (29% from Fat, 13% from Protein, 58% from Carb); 12 g Protein; 12 g Tot Fat; 3 g Sat Fat; 3 g Mono Fat; 54 g Carb; 6 g Fiber; 20 g Sugar; 186 mg Calcium; 3 mg Iron; 279 mg Sodium; 90 mg Cholesterol

Per Serving (2 egg whites): 347 Cal (26% from Fat, 13% from Protein, 61% from Carb); 12 g Protein; 10 g Tot Fat; 2 g Sat Fat; 2 g Mono Fat; 54 g Carb; 6 g Fiber; 20 g Sugar; 177 mg Calcium; 2 mg Iron; 289 mg Sodium; 8 mg Cholesterol

Scrambled Eggs with Mushrooms and Onions

serves 2

ingredients

1 teaspoon olive oil
1/2 small yellow onion, chopped
(about 2 ounces)
4 white mushrooms, sliced
(about 4 ounces)

1 garlic clove, minced
1 tablespoon freshly minced basil
4 eggs
1 tablespoon milk
Salt and pepper to taste

cooking instructions

Heat the oil in a nonstick pan over medium heat. Add the onion and sauté until translucent. Add the garlic, mushrooms, and sauté until mushrooms are cooked through. Beat the eggs with the milk in a bowl. Add the basil and season to taste. Pour the mixture over the vegetables. Cook over medium heat, stirring and scraping the bottom and sides of the pan constantly with a wooden spoon. As soon as the eggs begin to set, remove from heat, continue to stir for a few seconds, and serve immediately.

nutritional facts

Per Serving: 240 Cal (53% from Fat, 29% from Protein, 18% from Carb); 18 g Protein; 14 g Tot Fat; 4 g Sat Fat; 6 g Mono Fat; 11 g Carb; 1 g Fiber; 4 g Sugar; 106 mg Calcium; 3 mg Iron; 171 mg Sodium; 491 mg Cholesterol

Salmon and Asparagus Omelet

serves 2

ingredients

4 eggs
1 teaspoon canola oil
1/2 tablespoon water
3 ounces wild smoked salmon
4 asparagus spears, cooked
1/4 small onion, diced
(about 1 ounce)

1/2 small garlic clove, minced
A couple pinches of fresh dill, minced
Lemon juice to taste
Salt and pepper to taste

cooking instructions

Heat the oil in a nonstick pan over medium heat. Add the onions and sauté until translucent. Add the garlic, asparagus, lemon juice, and sauté for 2 minutes. Spread the vegetables evenly over the bottom of the pan.

In a bowl, beat the eggs, water, and season to taste. Add the egg mixture to the asparagus and let the eggs set. Add the smoked salmon and sprinkle the dill. Reduce heat and continue to cook for 2 to 3 minutes. Fold over in half, cook another minute, and serve immediately.

nutritional facts

Per Serving: 260 Cal (56% from Fat, 38% from Protein, 6% from Carb); 24 g Protein; 16 g Tot Fat; 4 g Sat Fat; 7 g Mono Fat; 4 g Carb; 1 g Fiber; 2 g Sugar; 97 mg Calcium; 4 mg Iron; 503 mg Sodium; 501 mg Cholesterol

Country Frittata

serves 2

ingredients

4 eggs
1 tablespoon water
1 teaspoon olive oil
1 green onion, chopped
1 garlic clove, minced
1 small zucchini, sliced
(about 4 ounces)

Half medium red bell pepper,
sliced (about 2 ounces)
1 tablespoon fresh salad herbs,
minced
Salt and pepper to taste

cooking instructions

Heat the oil in a nonstick pan over medium heat. Add the garlic, zucchini, and sauté for 2 to 3 minutes. Add the bell pepper, green onion, herbs, and continue to sauté for 2 minutes. Spread the vegetables evenly over the bottom of the pan. In a bowl, beat the eggs, water, and season to taste. Add the egg mixture to the vegetables and let the eggs set. Reduce heat and continue to cook for 2 to 3 minutes. Flip over and continue to cook until golden brown. Transfer to a platter, cut in wedges, and serve immediately.

Serving suggestion: Serve over a bed of fresh spinach.

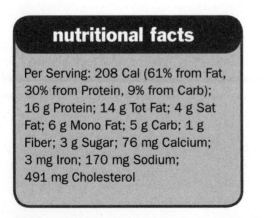

nutritional facts

Per Serving: 208 Cal (61% from Fat, 30% from Protein, 9% from Carb); 16 g Protein; 14 g Tot Fat; 4 g Sat Fat; 6 g Mono Fat; 5 g Carb; 1 g Fiber; 3 g Sugar; 76 mg Calcium; 3 mg Iron; 170 mg Sodium; 491 mg Cholesterol

Breakfast Shake

serves 1

ingredients

4 ounces pure Acai,
no sugar added
1 cup mixed berries
(about 4 ounces)
1 small banana, skin removed
(about 4 ounces)
1/2 cup natural apple juice
(no sugar added)

✓ *Acai is a fruit grown in the Amazon rain forest. It has a chocolaty flavor and is considered to be one of nature's healthiest foods. Due to its high concentration of antioxidants, anthocyanins (approximately 20 times the amount in red wine), amino acids, essential omegas, fibers and protein, it is a great addition to a healthy diet. If not available in your local store, check the Internet for this product.*

cooking instructions

Place all the ingredients in a blender and fill with ice. Puree on high speed until smooth. Divide between two tall glasses and serve immediately with a straw.

nutritional facts

Per Serving: 152 Cal (22% from Fat, 6% from Protein, 72% from Carb); 3 g Protein; 4 g Tot Fat; 1 g Sat Fat; 0 g Mono Fat; 30 g Carb; 5 g Fiber; 16 g Sugar; 20 mg Calcium; 1 mg Iron; 11 mg Sodium; 0 mg Cholesterol

Soup & Salad

Soups and salads are very versatile and can be served as an appetizer, main course, side dish, or even dessert. **They are quick and healthy meal options, and can be a great way to use leftovers.** In addition, salad recipes don't require much cooking, if any, and the techniques used are very basic. Salads taste better when put together at the last minute. They will be more appealing and pleasing with their fresh colors, textures, and flavors.

Here are a few important things to keep in mind whenever you prepare soups or salads.

First, stay away from croutons and avoid unhealthy salad dressings. Healthy dressing choices include oil (particularly olive oil, canola oil, avocado oil, flaxseed oil, and/or walnut oil unless you have a nut allergy, and vinegar (wine, balsamic, or apple) or citrus juices with fresh herbs. Apple cider vinegar can be beneficial to your health due to its cleansing and healing properties. So don't hesitate to substitute it for vinegar or citrus juice.

If you have no problems with nuts, use a few nuts in your salads such as walnuts, almonds, pistachios, hazelnuts, and pepitas, or sprinkle freshly ground flaxseeds. Include lots of vegetables in your salads, particularly the recommended greens and vegetables in the shopping list of this book, as they are very powerful antioxidants. **Onions, scallions, shallots, and garlic are also important, as they too have cancer-fighting properties and help lower bad cholesterol (LDL).**

Your salads may contain an adequate amount of protein, which should come from lean sources such as fish, poultry, or tofu. **Plant protein sources such as dry beans, lentils, and garbanzos may be substituted.** They will provide fibers and polyphenols which have good anti-inflammatory and anti-allergenic properties. Note: if you are not a vegetarian, try to maintain a good mix of animal and plant proteins to ensure you get the nutrients you need. **The addition of fresh herbs and freshly ground spices will add flavors and antioxidants which will help boost your immune system.** Limit cheeses to lower-fat brands to minimize fat intake. Shredding just a little fresh parmesan over a salad can add much flavor without adding unwanted calories. As for a soup, be careful not to overcook the vegetables you add to your soup bases, as they will lose their nutrients. This can be tricky because a soup's ingredients will continue to cook as long as the soup is hot, even after you've taken it off the stove. So undercook the vegetables to allow for that extra time and to preserve their nutritive values. For herbs in soup, use dry herbs at first and finish with fresh herbs (using fresh herbs at the beginning will only be a waste of money, as the flavors will evaporate during the cooking process.) For balanced nutrition, be sure to include lean proteins, complex carbohydrates, and vegetables just as you would in your salads.

Vegetable Soup

serves 6

ingredients

2 teaspoons canola oil
1 large onion, diced
(about 8 ounces)
1 small leek, chopped
(about 4 ounces)
1 large carrot, diced
(about 4 ounces)
2 large celery stalks, diced
(about 4 ounces)
1 large turnip, diced
(about 6 ounces)
1 medium red bell-pepper, diced
(about 6 ounces)
2 garlic cloves, minced

✔ *You can easily double this recipe and use it for a variety of meals, or freeze portions. Add brown rice, diced chicken, diced turkey, meatballs (made from ground turkey, venison, or buffalo), fish pieces, shellfish, or tofu.*

6 cups vegetable or chicken stock
(low fat and low-sodium)
1 bouquet garni
2 small fresh tomatoes (about 6 ounces)
1 bunch spinach, chopped
2 tablespoons freshly minced parsley
Salt and pepper

cooking instructions

Make a small X incision on the top and bottom of the tomatoes. Blanch the tomatoes for 20 seconds. Remove and place in ice-cold water to stop the cooking process. Peel, seed, and dice the tomatoes.

Heat the oil in a large pan over medium high heat. Add the onion and sauté until translucent. Add the leek, carrot, celery stalks, bell pepper, and sauté rapidly. Add the turnip, garlic, stock, bouquet garni, and bring to a boil. Reduce heat and simmer until barely tender. Add the tomatoes, spinach, and simmer for a minute. Finish with the parsley and adjust seasonings.

nutritional facts

Per Serving: 103 Cal (17% from Fat, 13% from Protein, 70% from Carb); 4 g Protein; 2 g Tot Fat; 0 g Sat Fat; 1 g Mono Fat; 20 g Carb; 5 g Fiber; 6 g Sugar; 113 mg Calcium; 3 mg Iron; 83 mg Sodium; 0 mg Cholesterol

Carrots and Apple Soup

serves 4

ingredients

5 large carrots, peeled and sliced
(about 20 ounces)
1 large Golden Delicious apple,
peeled and quartered (about 6
ounces)
1 medium onion, peeled and
quartered (about 6 ounces)

4 cups chicken stock
(low-fat and low-sodium)
1 bouquet garni
1/4 teaspoon ginger powder
Salt and pepper, to taste

cooking instructions

Place the carrots, apple, onion, stock, bouquet garni, and ginger
powder in a large pan. Bring to boil over medium heat. Reduce heat,
cover, and simmer until the vegetables are cooked through (about 10
to 15 minutes). Transfer to a blender and purée with enough liquid to
obtain a soup consistency. Season to taste
and serve immediately.

nutritional facts

Per Serving: 135 Cal (11% from Fat,
18% from Protein, 71% from Carb);
7 g Protein; 2 g Tot Fat; 0 g Sat Fat;
1 g Mono Fat; 26 g Carb; 5 g Fiber;
13 g Sugar; 68 mg Calcium;
1 mg Iron; 171 mg Sodium;
0 mg Cholesterol

Squash Soup

serves 4

ingredients

2 large zucchini, peeled and sliced (about 12 ounces)
2 large yellow squash, peeled and quartered (about 12 ounces)
1 medium onion, peeled and quartered (about 6 ounces)
3 ½ cups chicken stock (low-fat and low-sodium)

1 bouquet garni
4 tablespoons freshly minced basil
4 tablespoons low-fat plain Greek yogurt
Salt and pepper to taste

cooking instructions

Place the zucchini, squash, onion, stock, and bouquet garni in a large pan. Bring to boil over medium heat. Reduce heat, cover, and simmer until the vegetables are cooked through (about 10 to 15 minutes). Transfer to a blender and purée with enough liquid to obtain a soup consistency. Return to pan, add the basil, and season to taste. Bring to a boil and serve immediately. Top each serving with a tablespoon of yogurt.

nutritional facts

Per Serving: 135 Cal (11% from Fat, 18% from Protein, 71% from Carb); 7 g Protein; 2 g Tot Fat; 0 g Sat Fat; 1 g Mono Fat; 26 g Carb; 5 g Fiber; 13 g Sugar; 68 mg Calcium; 1 mg Iron; 171 mg Sodium; 0 mg Cholesterol

Lentil Soup with Ground Turkey

serves 4

ingredients

3 teaspoons canola oil
1 large onion, diced small
(about 8 ounces)
1 large carrot, diced small (about
4 ounces)
2 large celery stalks, diced small
(about 4 ounces)
2 garlic cloves, minced

6 cups chicken stock
(low-fat and low-sodium)
3 cups dried lentils
8 ounces ground turkey
1 bouquet garni
Salt and pepper

cooking instructions

Heat 2 teaspoons of oil in a large pan over high heat. Add the onion
and sauté until translucent. Add the carrot, celery, garlic, and cook for 2
minutes. Add the stock, lentils, bouquet garni, and bring to a boil. Reduce
heat, cover, and simmer for 35 minutes. Skim the surface as needed.
Continue to simmer uncovered for 10 minutes in order to thicken the
soup. Remove the bouquet garni. Heat 1 teaspoon of oil in a medium pan
over high heat. Add the ground turkey and sauté until cooked through
(about 3 to 4 minutes). Strain and disregard any fat. Add the meat to
the prepared lentils and bring to a boil. Adjust seasonings and serve
immediately.

If the soup turns out too thick,
adjust with stock. If the soup is
too thin, reduce the liquid more
or mash a little bit of the lentils
and return mixture to the pan.

nutritional facts

Per Serving: 262 Cal (19% from Fat,
39% from Protein, 42% from Carb);
26 g Protein; 6 g Tot Fat; 1 g Sat
Fat; 2 g Mono Fat; 28 g Carb;
9 g Fiber; 6 g Sugar; 87 mg Calcium;
5 mg Iron; 617 mg Sodium;
37 mg Cholesterol

Fish Soup

serves 8

✓ *For this soup, these fish work best: cod, bream, eel, haddock, hake, mackerel, monkfish, perch, red snapper, or white fish. Remember, the total calories will vary depending on the fish selected.*

ingredients

2 teaspoons olive oil
1 large onion, diced small
(about 8 ounces)
1 large carrot, diced small
(about 4 ounces)
5 garlic cloves, minced
6 ounces Chardonnay wine
(lemon and buttery tone)
4 pounds of various fish
(see note above)
6 cups fish stock
(low-fat and low-sodium)

1 bouquet garni
2 medium tomatoes
(about 8 ounces)
1/4 cup freshly minced parsley
2 large and long strip orange zests
4 saffron sprigs
1 teaspoon fennel seeds
2 large potatoes, peeled and
quartered (about one pound)
2 tablespoons freshly chopped
basil
Salt and pepper to taste

cooking instructions

Make a small X incision on the top and bottom of the tomatoes. Blanch the tomatoes for 20 seconds. Remove and place the tomatoes in ice-cold water to stop the cooking process. Peel, seed, and dice the tomatoes. Set aside.

Heat the oil in a large, deep pan over high heat. Add the onions and sauté until translucent. Add the carrots, garlic, and sauté for 2 minutes. Add the wine and reduce by half. Add the stock, bouquet garni, tomatoes, pars-ley, orange zest, saffron, fennel seeds, potatoes, and bring to a boil. Reduce heat and simmer for 10 minutes. Add the fish and simmer for another 10 minutes. Check for the doneness of the potatoes and fish. Remove the bouquet garni and orange zest. Skim the surface, adjust seasonings, and serve immediately.

nutritional facts

Per Serving: 384 Cal (19% from Fat, 15% from Protein, 65% from Carb); 15 g Protein; 8 g Tot Fat; 1 g Sat Fat; 2 g Mono Fat; 63 g Carb; 5 g Fiber; 25 g Sugar; 525 mg Calcium; 2 mg Iron; 132 mg Sodium; 5 mg Cholesterol

Roasted Tomato and Red Bell Pepper Soup

serves 4

> ✔ *Serve this soup cold in the summer for a refreshing taste.*

ingredients

2 teaspoons olive oil

5 large tomatoes, halved lengthwise (about 2 pounds)

3 large red bell peppers, seeded and quartered (about 24 ounces)

4 to 6 garlic cloves, peeled

1 teaspoon freshly minced thyme

2 tablespoons freshly minced basil

2 cups vegetable stock (low-fat and low-sodium)

Salt and pepper

cooking instructions

Preheat the oven to 450°F. Place the tomatoes, red bell peppers, and garlic on an oiled baking sheet. Drizzle a little olive oil over the vegetables and roast for 30 minutes or until brown. Remove from the oven and cool.

Puree the vegetables in a blender. Transfer to a saucepan; add the thyme, and enough stock to bring to a soup consistency. Add the basil and bring to a boil over medium heat. Adjust seasonings and serve immediately.

nutritional facts

Per Serving: 157 Cal (18% from Fat, 13% from Protein, 69% from Carb); 6 g Protein; 4 g Tot Fat; 1 g Sat Fat; 2 g Mono Fat; 31 g Carb; 5 g Fiber; 8 g Sugar; 100 mg Calcium; 2 mg Iron; 83 mg Sodium; 0 mg Cholesterol

Leek and Potato Soup

serves 4

✔ *For a different and healthy garnish, you can use shredded greens such as spinach, watercress, sorrel, or bok choy.*

ingredients

1 teaspoon canola oil
1 medium onion, diced
(about 6 ounces)
2 garlic cloves, minced
3 large leeks, white part only,
thinly sliced (about 12 ounces)
2 medium potatoes, thinly sliced
(about 12 ounces)

4 cups vegetable or chicken stock
(low-fat and low-sodium)
1 bouquet garni
Salt and pepper to taste
Freshly minced chives for garnish

cooking instructions

Heat the oil in a pan over medium high heat. Add the onion and sauté until translucent. Add the garlic, leeks, and sweat rapidly. Add the potatoes, stock, bouquet garni, and bring to boil. Reduce heat and simmer until the vegetables are tender and the potatoes cooked through. Remove the bouquet garni and pass the soup through a food mill. Use liquid as needed to obtain the right soup consistency. Season and serve immediately, garnished with the chives

nutritional facts

Per Serving: 237 Cal (13% from Fat, 9% from Protein, 78% from Carb); 6 g Protein; 3 g Tot Fat; 0 g Sat Fat; 2 g Mono Fat; 48 g Carb; 4 g Fiber; 9 g Sugar; 98 mg Calcium; 3 mg Iron; 845 mg Sodium; 0 mg Cholesterol

Black Bean Soup

serves 4

ingredients

2 teaspoons canola oil
1 large onion, diced small
(about 8 ounces)
1 large carrot, diced small
(about 4 ounces)
2 large celery stalks, diced small
(about 4 ounces)
2 garlic cloves, minced

6 cups vegetable or chicken stock
(low-fat and low-sodium)
12 ounces dried black beans,
rinsed
1 bouquet garni
Salt and pepper to taste

cooking instructions

Place the beans in a large pot and cover (way over) with water. Bring to a boil over high heat. Remove from heat and let soak for an hour. (Or, you may soak the beans overnight in cold water.) Strain and set aside.

Heat the oil in a large pan over high heat. Add the onion and sauté until translucent. Add the carrot, celery stalks, garlic, and cook for 2 minutes. Add the beans, bouquet garni, and bring to a boil. Reduce heat, cover, and simmer for 45 minutes or until tender. Skim the surface as needed. Remove 1/3 cup of the beans and puree with a fork. Mix the puree with the remaining soup. Remove the bouquet garni, adjust seasonings and serve immediately. If the soup is too thick, adjust with stock. If the soup is too thin, reduce the liquid more.

nutritional facts

Per Serving: 198 Cal (13% from Fat, 26% from Protein, 61% from Carb); 13 g Protein; 3 g Tot Fat; 0 g Sat Fat; 1 g Mono Fat; 31 g Carb; 10 g Fiber; 4 g Sugar; 86 mg Calcium; 3 mg Iron; 877 mg Sodium; 0 mg Cholesterol

Chickpea, Tomato, and Rice Soup

serves 4

ingredients

1 teaspoon olive oil
1 small onion, diced
(about 4 ounces)
8 ounces chopped Italian plum
tomatoes (can)
1/2 cup brown rice
12 ounces cooked chickpeas
3 garlic cloves, minced

5 cups chicken stock
1/2 teaspoon fresh rosemary,
minced
2 tablespoons fresh parsley,
chopped
Salt and pepper to taste

cooking instructions

Heat the oil in a large pan over high heat. Add the onion and sauté until translucent. Add the garlic, tomatoes, rosemary, and cook until the juices are evaporated. Add the rice, stock, and bring to boil. Reduce heat, cover, and simmer for 25 minutes. Add the chickpeas and continue to cook for 5 minutes, or until the rice is cooked through. Add the parsley, season to taste, and serve immediately.

nutritional facts

Per Serving: 391 Cal (15% from Fat, 22% from Protein, 64% from Carb); 22 g Protein; 6 g Tot Fat; 1 g Sat Fat; 2 g Mono Fat; 64 g Carb; 16 g Fiber; 12 g Sugar; 136 mg Calcium; 7 mg Iron; 719 mg Sodium; 0 mg Cholesterol

Tropical Gazpacho

serves 6

ingredients

1 ½ cup organic tomato juice
1 cup chopped mango
1 cup chopped papaya
1/2 cup chopped pineapple
1/2 cup chopped, seeded, peeled cucumber

1/2 cup chopped orange bell pepper
1/2 small red onion, peeled and chopped
1/8 cup freshly minced cilantro
Tabasco to taste (optional)
Salt and pepper to taste

cooking instructions

Puree the ingredients in a blender. Transfer to a large bowl and season to taste. Refrigerate and serve cold.

nutritional facts

Per Serving (8 ounces): 52 Cal (3% from Fat, 8% from Protein, 89% from Carb); 1 g Protein; 0 g Tot Fat; 0 g Sat Fat; 0 g Mono Fat; 13 g Carb; 2 g Fiber; 10 g Sugar; 22 mg Calcium;0 mg Iron; 169 mg Sodium; 0 mg Cholesterol

Beet Salad with Shaved Pecorino

serves 4

✓ *This salad may also be served with lettuce, endives, apples, or any combination of those.*

ingredients

2 large beets (about 20 ounces)
1/4 cup walnuts, chopped
2 tablespoons walnut oil
1 lemon
1 tablespoon shaved Pecorino cheese
Salt and pepper to taste

cooking instructions

Place the beets in a large pan and cover with water. Bring to boil over high heat. Reduce heat, cover, and simmer for 30 minutes, or until tender. Strain and cool. Peel and slice the beets. Place the slices overlapping each other in a serving platter. Season the beets with salt and pepper. Drizzle with the oil and a little lemon juice. Evenly spread the cheese and serve immediately.

nutritional facts

Per Serving: 181 Cal (56% from Fat, 9% from Protein, 35% from Carb); 4 g Protein; 12 g Tot Fat; 1 g Sat Fat; 2 g Mono Fat; 18 g Carb; 6 g Fiber; 10 g Sugar; 64 mg Calcium; 2 mg Iron; 135 mg Sodium; 1 mg Cholesterol

Four Bean Salad

serves 6

> ✔ *This salad may be served with lettuce, tomato, and avocado. You may substitute one 15–ounce can cooked beans for each dried bean. Rinse before use.*

ingredients

For the salad:
4 ounces dried garbanzo beans
4 ounces dried black beans
4 ounces dried red beans
4 ounces green beans
1/4 small red onion, diced
(about 1 ounce)

For the dressing:
1 large garlic clove, minced
2 tablespoons olive oil
4 tablespoons cider vinegar
2 tablespoons fresh salad herbs, minced
Salt and pepper to taste

cooking instructions

For the dressing: In a bowl mix the garlic, oil, vinegar, and herbs.

For the salad: Cook the beans separately, following the package instructions. Generally, it takes about 30 to 45 minutes to cook these types of beans. Place the green beans with a little salt in a pan and bring to boil over high heat. Cook until desired tenderness. Strain and place immediately in ice-cold water to stop the cooking process. Strain and pat dry. Place all the beans and red onion in a large bowl. Add the dressing, season to taste, and refrigerate for an hour before serving.

nutritional facts

Per Serving: 245 Cal (22% from Fat, 20% from Protein, 58% from Carb); 13 g Protein; 6 g Tot Fat; 1 g Sat Fat; 4 g Mono Fat; 37 g Carb; 12 g Fiber; 4 g Sugar; 79 mg Calcium; 4 mg Iron; 12 mg Sodium; 0 mg Cholesterol

Greek Salad with Cod Fish

serves 4

ingredients

Four 4-ounce cooked cod fillets
4 cups mixed greens
1 large cucumber, skin removed,
seeded, and sliced
(about 12 ounces)
2 large tomatoes, sliced
(about 12 ounces)
1/2 small red onion, sliced
(about 2 ounces)

1 medium red bell pepper, sliced
(about 6 ounces)
1/4 cup black olives
4 tablespoons feta cheese
4 tablespoons Greek salad
dressing or vinaigrette
1 teaspoon freshly
minced oregano
Salt and pepper to taste

cooking instructions

Mix the vinaigrette with the oregano and set aside. Divide the mixed greens, cucumber, tomatoes, red onion, red bell pepper, black olives, and feta cheese among 4 plates. Top with the fish filet and season to taste. Sprinkle the vinaigrette and serve immediately.

nutritional facts

Per Serving: 222 Cal (33% from Fat, 43% from Protein, 24% from Carb); 24 g Protein; 8 g Tot Fat; 2 g Sat Fat; 2 g Mono Fat; 13 g Carb; 3 g Fiber; 6 g Sugar; 121 mg Calcium; 2 mg Iron; 505 mg Sodium; 57 mg Cholesterol

Quinoa and Apricot Salad

serves 4

ingredients

1 cup Quinoa
2 teaspoons olive oil
1 small red onion, diced
(about 4 ounces)
2 mushrooms, diced
(about 2 ounces)
1 tablespoon minced
fresh ginger root
1 small green jalapeno, minced

1 teaspoon turmeric
1 teaspoon coriander
1/4 teaspoon ground cinnamon
3 apricots, diced
1/4 cup chopped almonds
2 tablespoons freshly minced
parsley or mint
1 lemon

cooking instructions

Place a coffee filter into a fine mesh sieve. Rinse the Quinoa under cold water through the filter.

Heat the oil in a saucepan over medium heat. Add the Quinoa and sauté for a few minutes to lightly brown. Add the onion, mushrooms, ginger, jalapeno, and sauté for a minute or two. Add the turmeric, coriander, cinnamon, and season to taste. Add 2 cups of water or stock and bring to a boil. Reduce heat and simmer for 20 minutes or until the liquid is completely absorbed. Transfer the Quinoa to a bowl and drizzle with a little olive oil and lemon juice. Add the diced apricots, herbs, and almonds. Adjust seasoning and serve immediately.

nutritional facts

Per Serving: 274 Cal (35% from Fat, 11% from Protein, 53% from Carb); 8 g Protein; 11 g Tot Fat; 1 g Sat Fat; 7 g Mono Fat; 39 g Carb; 6 g Fiber; 3 g Sugar; 72 mg Calcium; 5 mg Iron; 13 mg Sodium; 0 mg Cholesterol

Grapefruit and Crabmeat Salad

serves 2

ingredients

1 large pink grapefruit
(about 16 ounces grapefruit)
Two 4-ounce crabmeat portions
(without excess water)
2 tablespoons low-fat canola
mayonnaise

1 cup lettuce, shredded
1 tablespoon freshly minced
cilantro
1 lime
Chili powder to taste
Salt and pepper

cooking instructions

Place the crabmeat in a bowl. Cut the grapefruit in half. Insert a thin
knife all around the skin to loosen up the flesh. Separate the flesh from
the skin and place it on a cutting board. Dice the flesh small and transfer
to the crabmeat bowl. Add mayonnaise, cilantro, a little lime juice, chili
powder, and season to taste. Cover with plastic wrap and refrigerate for
half an hour.

Equally divide the lettuce in two plates and top with the prepared
grapefruit crabmeat salad.

nutritional facts

Per Serving: 219 Cal (19% from Fat,
43% from Protein, 38% from Carb);
24 g Protein; 5 g Tot Fat; 1 g Sat
Fat; 1 g Mono Fat; 21 g Carb;
3 g Fiber; 16 g Sugar; 105 mg Calcium; 1 mg Iron; 1240 mg Sodium;
63 mg Cholesterol

Salmon and Vegetable Carpaccio

serves 2

ingredients

6 ounces thinly sliced wild
smoked salmon
1 medium cucumber, peeled
(about 8 ounces)
1 large yellow squash, peeled
(about 8 ounces)

2 green onions, minced
2 teaspoons fresh dill, minced
4 tablespoons olive oil
1 lemon
Salt and pepper to taste

cooking instructions

Remove a couple of zest strips from the lemon and mince. Juice the
lemon and set aside in a bowl. Add the olive oil, 1 teaspoon dill, half of
the prepared zest, and season to taste.

Thinly slice the cucumber and yellow squash. Refrigerate until use.
Equally divide the salmon in two plates, season to taste, and sprinkle
with dill. Pour half the dressing over and refrigerate for 20 minutes. In
the center of the salmon slices and in a round formation, alternate the
cucumber and squash slices. Season lightly and garnish with the green
onions, remaining zest and dill. Pour over the remaining dressing and
serve immediately.

nutritional facts

Per Serving: 388 Cal (69% from Fat,
18% from Protein, 13% from Carb);
19 g Protein; 31 g Tot Fat; 5 g Sat
Fat; 22 g Mono Fat; 14 g Carb; 5 g
Fiber; 4 g Sugar; 104 mg Calcium;
3 mg Iron; 687 mg Sodium; 20 mg
Cholesterol

Chicken Salad with Fruit

serves 4

ingredients

For the salad:
5 ounces fresh baby spinach
8 ounces cooked chicken breasts
(without skin), diced
2 avocados, diced
6 ounces red grapes
1 orange, wedged
1 mango, diced
4 teaspoons sliced almonds

For the dressing:
2 tablespoons olive oil
2 tablespoons lemon juice
1 tablespoon fresh salad herbs
Pinch of each curry and ginger
Salt and pepper to taste

cooking instructions

For the dressing: In a bowl mix the oil, lemon, and herbs. Blend in the curry, ginger, and season to taste.

For the salad: In a bowl mix the spinach, chicken, and the dressing. Add the fruits, avocados, and almonds.

nutritional facts

Per Serving: 376 Cal (51% from Fat, 17% from Protein, 32% from Carb); 17 g Protein; 22 g Tot Fat; 3 g Sat Fat; 15 g Mono Fat; 32 g Carb; 9 g Fiber; 19 g Sugar; 89 mg Calcium; 2 mg Iron; 75 mg Sodium; 33 mg Cholesterol

Niçoise Salad

serves 4

ingredients

For the salad:
5 ounces mesclun
6 ounces canned tuna in water, strained
2 large tomatoes, seeded and diced
1 yellow bell pepper, seeded, ribs removed, and julienned
1 small cucumber, peeled and sliced
1/2 cup cooked green beans (about 4 ounces)

4 tablespoons small niçoise black olives
4 anchovies
4 eggs

For the dressing:
1 shallot, minced
1 garlic clove, minced
3 tablespoons lemon juice
3 tablespoons olive oil
2 tablespoons salad herbs
Salt and pepper to taste

cooking instructions

For the dressing: In a bowl mix the shallot, garlic, lemon juice, oil, 1 tablespoon of herbs, and season to taste.

For the salad: Place the eggs in a pan, cover with water, add 2 teaspoons salt, and bring to a boil over medium heat. Reduce heat and simmer for 10 minutes. Remove the eggs and place them in cold water. Peel, quarter, and set aside.

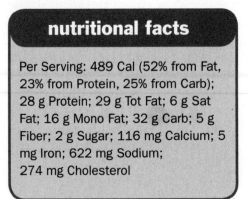

nutritional facts

Per Serving: 489 Cal (52% from Fat, 23% from Protein, 25% from Carb); 28 g Protein; 29 g Tot Fat; 6 g Sat Fat; 16 g Mono Fat; 32 g Carb; 5 g Fiber; 2 g Sugar; 116 mg Calcium; 5 mg Iron; 622 mg Sodium; 274 mg Cholesterol

In a large bowl mix the mesclun with half of the dressing. Add the tomatoes, bell pepper, cucumber, and green beans. Top with the tuna, eggs, anchovies, olives, and sprinkle the remaining herbs. Drizzle the remaining dressing and serve immediately.

Sugar Snap Peas and Tuna Salad

serves 4

ingredients

For the salad:
4 ounces mesclun
1 ½ can of tuna in water, strained
(9 ounces)
1 large carrot, thinly sliced
(about 4 ounces)
2 large tomatoes, seeded and
diced
1cup fresh sugar snap peas
(about 4 ounces)
Salt and pepper to taste

For the dressing:
1 shallot, minced
1 garlic clove, minced
3 tablespoons lemon juice
3 tablespoons olive oil
2 tablespoons salad herbs
Salt and pepper to taste

cooking instructions

Heat a steamer and add the sugar snap peas. Cook for 2 minutes. Add the carrots and continue to steam for 2 minutes or until desired doneness. In a bowl, mix the shallot, garlic, lemon juice, oil, 1 tablespoon of herbs, and season to taste. In a large bowl mix the mesclun with half of the dressing. Add the tuna, tomatoes, carrot slices, and sugar snap peas. Sprinkle with the remaining herbs and dressing before serving.

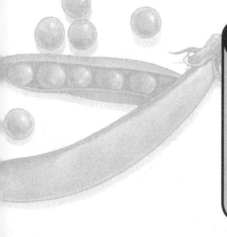

nutritional facts

Per Serving: 154 Cal (13% from Fat, 47% from Protein, 39% from Carb); 19 g Protein; 2 g Tot Fat; 1 g Sat Fat; 1 g Mono Fat; 15 g Carb; 4 g Fiber; 6 g Sugar; 63 mg Calcium; 2 mg Iron; 62 mg Sodium; 27 mg Cholesterol

Chicken Salad with Celery and Apple

serves 4

ingredients

For the salad:
1 large Romaine heart leaves, chopped (about 6 ounces)
12 ounces cooked chicken breasts, diced
2 large apples (about 12 ounces)
2 large celery stalks, diced (about 4 ounces)
1/4 cup walnuts, chopped
1 lemon

For the vinaigrette:
2 tablespoons cider vinegar
1 tablespoon lemon juice
2 teaspoons honey
1 tablespoon walnut oil
2 tablespoons olive oil
2 tablespoons fresh parsley, chopped
Salt and pepper to taste

cooking instructions

For the vinaigrette: In a large bowl mix the vinegar, 1 tablespoon lemon juice, honey, oil, parsley, and season to taste.

For the salad: Peel, core, and dice the apples. Mix them with some lemon juice to prevent browning. In a bowl place the romaine, chicken, apples, and celery. Mix in the dressing, add the walnuts, and serve immediately.

nutritional facts

Per Serving: 304 Cal (49% from Fat, 24% from Protein, 26% from Carb); 20 g Protein; 18 g Tot Fat; 3 g Sat Fat; 8 g Mono Fat; 21 g Carb; 5 g Fiber; 13 g Sugar; 61 mg Calcium; 2 mg Iron; 83 mg Sodium; 55 mg Cholesterol

Lentil Salad

serves 6

ingredients

For the salad:
1 pound lentils
1 tablespoon garlic cloves, minced
1 bouquet garni
1 bay leaf
1 orange, juiced

For the dressing:
2 tablespoons wine vinegar
1 tablespoon shallot, minced
1 teaspoon Dijon mustard
6 tablespoons walnut oil
3 tablespoons freshly minced salad herbs
Salt and pepper to taste

cooking instructions

For the dressing: In a bowl mix the vinegar, shallot, and mustard. Slowly whisk in the oil. Add the herbs and season to taste.

For the salad: Rinse the lentils and place them in a pan. Add enough water to completely cover them. Bring to a boil over high heat. Remove from heat and set aside covered for 1 hour.

Strain and place in the large pan. Add water (3 times the volume of the lentils), garlic, bay leaf, and bouquet garni. Bring to a boil over high heat. Reduce heat, cover, and simmer for 20 to 25 minutes, or until tender.

Remove the bouquet garni and bay leaf. Strain the lentils and transfer to a bowl. Mix in the vinaigrette and refrigerate for 30 minutes. Serve cold.

nutritional facts

Per Serving: 230 Cal (53% from Fat, 12% from Protein, 35% from Carb); 7 g Protein; 14 g Tot Fat; 2 g Sat Fat; 6 g Mono Fat; 21 g Carb; 7 g Fiber; 2 g Sugar; 40 mg Calcium; 3 mg Iron; 12 mg Sodium; 0 mg Cholesterol

Tomato and Basil Salad

serves 4

> ✓ *You may shred a little parmesan cheese once individually served.*

ingredients

6 large tomatoes (about 2 pounds)
1 shallot, minced
1 large garlic clove, minced
3 tablespoons olive oil
1 tablespoon flaxseed oil
(or olive oil, if unavailable)

2 tablespoons balsamic vinegar
(preferably aged)
6 to 8 fresh basil leaves
1 tablespoon fresh parsley,
minced
Salt and pepper to taste

cooking instructions

Mince half the basil and shred the remaining half. Disregard each end of the tomatoes. Slice the tomatoes and spread them over a platter. Sprinkle with a little salt and set aside for 20 minutes.

In a bowl mix the shallot, garlic, vinegar, and whisk in the oils. Add the minced basil, parsley, and season to taste.

Transfer the tomatoes to another serving platter. Spread the remaining basil, pour over the dressing, and serve immediately.

nutritional facts

Per Serving: 172 Cal (70% from Fat,
5% from Protein, 25% from Carb); 2
g Protein; 14 g Tot Fat; 2 g Sat Fat;
8 g Mono Fat; 12 g Carb; 3 g Fiber;
0 g Sugar; 17 mg Calcium;
1 mg Iron; 22 mg Sodium;
0 mg Cholesterol

Fish/Seafood Entrées

A healthy diet includes plenty of fish. Why? **Fish are sources of proteins, fats, vitamins, and minerals, as well as many essential amino acids.** In addition, one of the best sources for Omega-3 fatty acids are oily fish like cod, tuna, salmon, sardines, herring, and mackerel—and all are easier to digest than meat.

You may have already heard about the health benefits of Omega-3 fatty acids, which help promote weight loss while still having a positive effect on the metabolizing of muscle proteins. Omega-3 fatty acids also help **reduce inflammation and lower bad cholesterol (LDL)**. As for shellfish, keep in mind that the protein levels are usually a little lower than fish and, from a nutrition standpoint, can result in higher cholesterol. So be careful not to over-indulge in shellfish.

Cooking fish and shellfish requires particular attention, as the flesh tends to be rather delicate. It is recommended that you use cooking techniques such as steaming, baking, broiling, barbecuing, or sautéing in a nonstick pan with very little oil.

Ahi Tartar

serves 4

ingredients

Four 4-ounce Ahi fillets
4 tablespoons shallots, chopped
1 medium cucumber
(about 8 ounces)
2 lemons
2 limes
1 medium red bell pepper,
seeded and ribs removed, diced
(about 6 ounces)

2 jalapeno chiles, seeded and
diced
1 sage leaf
4 tablespoons basil, chopped
1 teaspoon green tea
1 teaspoon honey
2 tablespoons olive oil
2 cups baby mixed greens
Salt and pepper to taste

cooking instructions

Make nice strips of the lemon and lime zests. Mince and set aside. Juice
the lemon, lime, and set aside. Cut the cucumber in half and remove
seeds. Cut into half again and dice. On low heat, warm the lemon juice,
lime juice, tea powder, sage, and honey until the honey is well incorporated. Remove and cool down. Refrigerate until cold.

Dice the Ahi, place it into a soup plate and season to taste. Mix in the
shallot, cucumber, red bell pepper, jalapeno chiles, and basil. Drizzle with
the olive oil, add the cold marinade, and refrigerate for 20 to 30 minutes.

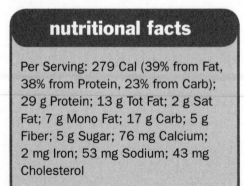

Equally divide the baby greens
among two ice-cold plates.
With a slotted spoon, scoop out
the Ahi Tartar. Drizzle with a
little bit of the marinade and
serve immediately.

nutritional facts

Per Serving: 279 Cal (39% from Fat,
38% from Protein, 23% from Carb);
29 g Protein; 13 g Tot Fat; 2 g Sat
Fat; 7 g Mono Fat; 17 g Carb; 5 g
Fiber; 5 g Sugar; 76 mg Calcium;
2 mg Iron; 53 mg Sodium; 43 mg
Cholesterol

Tuna Spanish Style

serves 4

ingredients

Four 5-ounce tuna fillets
1 tablespoon olive oil
2 large onions, sliced
(about 1 pound)
6 large tomatoes
(about 2 pounds)
1 large green bell pepper; ribs
and seeds removed, sliced
(about 8 ounces)

1 tablespoon wheat flour
3 garlic cloves, minced
1 pinch dry thyme
1 pinch dry oregano
2 tablespoons fresh parsley,
minced
1/2 cup brown rice
Salt and pepper to taste

cooking instructions

Cook the rice according to package instructions. Make a small X incision on the top and bottom of the tomatoes. Blanch the tomatoes for 20 seconds. Place in ice-cold water to stop the cooking process. Peel, seed, and dice the tomatoes.

Heat 2 teaspoons of olive oil in a deep nonstick pan over high heat. Add the onions and sauté until translucent. Add the garlic, bell pepper, thyme, oregano, and sauté for 3 minutes over medium heat. Sprinkle with the flour and mix well. Add the tomatoes and continue to cook for 3 to 4 minutes.

Meanwhile, heat the remaining oil in a nonstick skillet over high heat. Add the fish and brown on both sides. Slide the fish into the vegetables, cover, and continue to cook for 15 to 20 minutes over low heat.

Transfer the fish to a serving platter. If necessary, thicken the sauce over medium heat. Add to the fish and serve immediately with the rice.

nutritional facts

Per Serving: 443 Cal (26% from Fat, 35% from Protein, 39% from Carb); 39 g Protein; 13 g Tot Fat; 3 g Sat Fat; 6 g Mono Fat; 44 g Carb; 6 g Fiber; 7 g Sugar; 70 mg Calcium; 3 mg Iron; 85 mg Sodium; 54 mg Cholesterol

Broiled Salmon with Dill

serves 4

> ✓ *This fish goes well with the Marinated Vegetables with Lemon (see page 112) and lemon wedges.*

ingredients

Four 5-ounce salmon fillets
1 tablespoon olive oil
4 to 5 fresh dill branches, minced
Salt and pepper to taste

cooking instructions

Preheat the broiler. Rub olive oil over the flesh side of the fillets. Lightly season the fillets and spread the minced dill over them. Place the fillets on a greased pan, skin side up. Brush olive oil over the skin and broil for 3 to 4 minutes. Turn over and continue to broil for a few minutes or until the salmon flesh start to flake.

nutritional facts

Per Serving: 295 Cal (57% from Fat, 39% from Protein, 4% from Carb); 29 g Protein; 19 g Tot Fat; 4 g Sat Fat; 8 g Mono Fat; 3 g Carb; 1 g Fiber; 0 g Sugar; 34 mg Calcium; 1 mg Iron; 85 mg Sodium; 84 mg Cholesterol

Salmon with Orange Sauce

serves 4

ingredients

Four 5-ounce salmon fillets
1 teaspoon canola oil
1 shallot, thinly sliced
2 oranges
1 teaspoon coriander seeds, crushed
1 1/2 cup fresh orange juice
1 tablespoon orange blossom honey

1 teaspoon dry parsley
Cornstarch with a little water
Salt and pepper to taste

For the vegetables:
2 pounds asparagus, trimmed
(about 32 asparagus, trimmed)
1/2 orange, juiced
Salt and pepper to taste

cooking instructions

Preheat the oven to 400 degrees F. For the fish: Julienne the orange zests and blanch them in boiling water for 2 minutes. Remove and set aside for later use. Remove the white outer part from the oranges. Slice the oranges (into approximately 3/8-inch slices).

Grease the bottom of a baking pan. Add the salmon and season to taste. Cover the fillets with a pinch of crushed coriander seeds, half of the zests, shallots, and the oranges slices. Warm up 1/4 cup orange juice with the remaining coriander seeds. Pour in the fish pan, cover with aluminum foil, and bake for 20 minutes, or until the flesh start to flake. Transfer the fish and accompaniment to a serving platter. Cover with aluminum foil to keep warm. Place the cooking liquid in a saucepan. Add the remaining zests, orange juice, and honey. Bring to a boil and reduce to 3/4 cup. Thicken with a little cornstarch mixed with water. Strain and return to the pan. Add parsley and season to taste. Pour the sauce over the fish. *For the vegetables:* Preheat a steamer. Add the asparagus and cook for 2 to 3 minutes or until desired doneness. Transfer the asparagus to a serving plate, sprinkle with a little orange juice, and season to taste. Serve the salmon with the asparagus.

nutritional facts

Per Serving: 461 Cal (36% from Fat, 31% from Protein, 34% from Carb); 36 g Protein; 19 g Tot Fat; 4 g Sat Fat; 7 g Mono Fat; 39 g Carb; 8 g Fiber; 24 g Sugar; 137 mg Calcium; 3 mg Iron; 125 mg Sodium; 88 mg Cholesterol

Steamed Salmon with Fennel

serves 4

ingredients

1 large salmon fillet (20 ounces)
1 medium onion, sliced
(about 6 ounces)
1 large carrot, sliced
(about 4 ounces)
1 teaspoon herbs de Provence
1/4 cup vegetables stock
(low-fat and low-sodium)
1 teaspoon fennel seeds
Salt and pepper to taste

For the vegetables:
1 tablespoon olive oil
2 large fennel bulbs, trimmed and
sliced (about 1 1/2 pound)
1 medium onion, sliced
(about 6 ounces)
1 tablespoon garlic cloves,
minced
1/4 cup vegetable stock
(low-fat and low-sodium)
Pinch cayenne pepper
Salt and pepper to taste

cooking instructions

Preheat the oven to 400 degrees F.

For the fish: Prepare a large aluminum foil. Place the salmon in the middle. Sprinkle over a little salt, some pepper, and the herbs de Provence. Top with the onion, carrot, and a few fennel slices (see vegetables). Fold the aluminum foil a bit; add the stock, and fennel seeds. Close and place on a baking dish. Bake for 25 to 30 minutes, or until the salmon flesh starts to flake.

For the vegetables: Heat the oil in a nonstick pan over high heat. Add the onion and sauté until translucent. Add the fennel slices, garlic, and sauté for 2 minutes. Pour in the vegetable stock, cover, and cook for 15 to 20 minutes over low heat. Add the cayenne pepper and season to taste.

Place the salmon in a serving platter with its vegetables and juices, and serve immediately with the fennel.

nutritional facts

Per Serving: 408 Cal (43% from Fat, 31% from Protein, 25% from Carb); 32 g Protein; 19 g Tot Fat; 4 g Sat Fat; 8 g Mono Fat; 26 g Carb; 8 g Fiber; 5 g Sugar; 144 mg Calcium; 2 mg Iron; 204 mg Sodium; 84 mg Cholesterol

Salmon with Basil Aioli

serves 4

ingredients

For the aioli:
6 to 8 large garlic cloves
1 teaspoon salt
2/3 cup olive oil
2 tablespoons fresh basil, minced

For the fish:
Four 5-ounce salmon fillets
2 teaspoons olive oil
Salt and pepper to taste

For the vegetables:
12 ounces baby carrots
1 large head broccoli florets
(about 12 ounces)
1 lemon, quartered
Salt and pepper to taste

cooking instructions

Preheat the broiler.

For the Aioli: All the ingredients must be at room temperature for the emulsion to take. In a food processor purée the garlic and salt to obtain a smooth paste. Pour in a drop of oil and mix until well incorporated. Continue the same way until most of the oil is incorporated. Please note: If you add the oil too quickly, the emulsion will not occur. Before adding the last drop of oil, blend in the basil and add a pinch of pepper.

For the fish: Place the salmon fillets on a greased baking pan. Brush olive oil over the fillets and sprinkle with pepper. Broil 3 to 4 minutes. Turn over, brush oil, sprinkle with pepper, and continue to broil for 3 to 4 minutes or until the flesh starts to flake. Transfer to a serving platter and sprinkle with salt to taste.

For the vegetables: Preheat a steamer. Add the carrots and cook for 4 minutes. Add the broccoli and continue to cook for 2 minutes. Transfer to a serving plate and season to taste. Serve the salmon and vegetables with the aioli.

nutritional facts

Per Serving: 608 Cal (69% from Fat, 20% from Protein, 11% from Carb); 32 g Protein; 48 g Tot Fat; 7 g Sat Fat; 31 g Mono Fat; 17 g Carb; 7 g Fiber; 5 g Sugar; 120 mg Calcium; 3 mg Iron; 734 mg Sodium; 78 mg Cholesterol

Cod Fish with Leek Fondue

serves 4

ingredients

Four 5-ounce cod fish fillets
5 medium leeks
(about 1 1/2 pounds)
1 tablespoon canola oil
1/4 cup vegetable stock
(low-fat and low-sodium)
1 tablespoon Dijon mustard
2 tablespoons crème fraiche
2 tablespoons lemon juice

2 tablespoons fresh chives,
minced
Salt and pepper to taste

For the vegetables:
3 medium potatoes, peeled and
quartered (about 1 pound)
3 large yellow squash, sliced in
1 inch pieces (about 1 pound)
Salt and pepper to taste

cooking instructions

Cut and discard the green part of the leeks. Cut the white part in half
and julienne. Wash well to remove any dirt and pat dry. Heat the oil in
a large sauté pan over high heat. Add the leeks and sauté for 2 minutes.
Add the stock and spread the leeks on the bottom of the pan. Place the
fish on top and sprinkle with pepper. Cover and cook for 20 minutes over
low heat. Meanwhile preheat the steamer. Add the potatoes and cook for
15 minutes. Add the squash and continue to cook for 5 minutes.

Remove the fish and set aside in a serving platter. Cover with aluminum foil to keep warm. Add the lemon juice, mustard, crème fraiche, and chives to the leeks. Mix well, adjust seasonings, and reduce for 2 minutes. Pour the sauce over the fish and serve immediately with the vegetables.

nutritional facts

Per Serving: 397 Cal (12% from Fat,
36% from Protein, 51% from Carb);
36 g Protein; 5 g Tot Fat; 1 g Sat
Fat; 2 g Mono Fat; 52 g Carb; 10 g
Fiber; 6 g Sugar; 115 mg Calcium; 4
mg Iron; 148 mg Sodium;
61 mg Cholesterol

Red Snapper en Papilotte

serves 4

ingredients

4 teaspoons olive oil
Four 5-ounce red snapper fillets
2 shallots, sliced
2 teaspoons lemon zest
4 tablespoons lemon juice
2 garlic cloves, minced
4 teaspoons parsley, minced

4 teaspoons capers
2 cups broccoli
2 cups yellow squash
Salt and pepper to taste

cooking instructions

Preheat the oven to 400° F. Prepare four aluminum foil packets. Place each red snapper fillet in the middle and season lightly. Equally divide and add the lemon zest, garlic, parsley, and capers. Drizzle with 1 teaspoon olive oil and 1 tablespoon lemon juice per portion. Fold the foils and place on a cookie sheet. Bake for 10 to 15 minutes or until the fish starts to flake.

Meanwhile preheat a steamer. Add the broccoli, yellow squash, and steam for 2 to 3 minutes, or until desired doneness. Serve immediately with the papilottes

nutritional facts

Per Serving: 268 Cal (23% from Fat, 50% from Protein, 27% from Carb); 34 g Protein; 7 g Tot Fat; 1 g Sat Fat; 1 g Mono Fat; 19 g Carb; 4 g Fiber; 5 g Sugar; 139 mg Calcium; 2 mg Iron; 212 mg Sodium; 52 mg Cholesterol

Halibut Provençale Style

serves 4

> ✓ *If herbs de Provence are unavailable, substitute Italian herbs.*

ingredients

Four 5-ounce halibut steaks
1 tablespoon olive oil
6 large tomatoes
(about 2 pounds)
1 large onion, sliced
(about 8 ounces)
1 large green bell pepper, seeded,
ribs removed, and sliced
(about 8 ounces)

1 large yellow bell pepper, seeded,
ribs removed, and sliced
(about 8 ounces)
2 tablespoons garlic cloves,
minced
2 pinches herbs de Provence
1 bunch fresh basil, shredded
1/2 cup wild rice
Salt and pepper to taste

cooking instructions

Make a small X incision on the top and bottom of the tomatoes. Blanch the tomatoes for 20 seconds. Remove and place in ice-cold water to stop the cooking process. Peel, seed, and slice the tomatoes.

Cook the wild rice according to package instructions. Heat the oil in a large pan over high heat. Add the halibut and brown. Turn over and cook for 2 minutes. Remove the fish and set aside on a plate. Deglaze the pan with a little water and swirl around to dissolve cooked particles on the bottom or side of the pan. Add the onion and cook for 2 minutes. Add the garlic, tomatoes, bell peppers, herbs de Provence, and sauté for 2 minutes. Slide in the fish fillets, cover, and cook for 15 to 20 minutes over low heat. Remove the fillets and set aside in a platter. Cover with aluminum foil to keep warm. Mix the basil with the vegetables and season to taste. Pour over the fish and serve immediately with the wild rice.

nutritional facts

Per Serving: 418 Cal (20% from Fat, 41% from Protein, 39% from Carb); 43 g Protein; 9 g Tot Fat; 1 g Sat Fat; 4 g Mono Fat; 42 g Carb; 6 g Fiber; 4 g Sugar; 134 mg Calcium; 4 mg Iron; 125 mg Sodium; 58 mg Cholesterol

Ocean Perch with Bell Pepper Coulis

serves 4

ingredients

Four 5-ounce ocean perch fillets
2 tablespoons olive oil
3 large red bell peppers
(about 1 pound)
1 shallot, minced
1 teaspoon garlic cloves, minced
1 teaspoon lemon juice

1 tablespoon fresh basil, chopped
Salt and pepper to taste

For the vegetables:
3 large eggplants, sliced medium
(about 2 pounds)
2 tablespoons olive oil
Salt and pepper to taste

cooking instructions

Preheat the broiler. For the fish: Place the red bell peppers on a baking sheet and char on all sides. If you have a gas stovetop, you may char the bell peppers over the flames. Once blackened on all sides, place in a paper bag and seal. Let stand for 10 minutes. Peel and seed the bell peppers. Remove ribs and quarter. Purée in a blender with the shallots, garlic, 1 tablespoon olive oil, basil, and lemon juice. Thin out with a little water and season to taste.

Heat 1 tablespoon of olive oil in a nonstick pan over medium heat. Add the fillets and brown. Turn over and continue to cook for 2 minutes. Add a little coulis, cover, reduce heat, and continue to cook until the flesh starts to flake. Transfer the fillets to a serving platter. Cover with aluminum foil to keep warm. Add the remaining coulis and bring to a boil over medium heat. Adjust seasonings and pour over the fillets.

For the vegetables: Brush the eggplant slices with olive oil, season to taste, and brown under the broiler on both sides. Time will vary depending on the thickness, make sure to keep a close eye on the eggplant. Remove and place on a serving platter. Serve the fillets with the eggplant slices.

nutritional facts

Per Serving: 335 Cal (41% from Fat, 36% from Protein, 24% from Carb); 31 g Protein; 16 g Tot Fat; 2 g Sat Fat; 10 g Mono Fat; 20 g Carb; 10 g Fiber; 10 g Sugar; 145 mg Calcium; 2 mg Iron; 95 mg Sodium; 128 mg Cholesterol

Shark with Ginger and Lime

serves 4

ingredients

Four 5-ounces shark fillets
1 tablespoon olive oil
1/2 small onion, diced
(about 2 ounces)
1 teaspoon garlic cloves, minced
1/2 cup vegetable stock
(low-fat and low-sodium)
1/2 cup lime juice
1 tablespoon honey
1 tablespoon fresh ginger, minced

2 tablespoons fresh parsley,
minced
1 teaspoon fresh rosemary
Cornstarch with a little water
Salt and pepper to taste

For the vegetables:
2 pounds chard, kale, spinach,
beet greens, or mustard greens;
cleaned and pat dry
1 lime
Salt and pepper to taste

cooking instructions

For the vegetables: Preheat a steamer. Add the greens and cook for 3 to 4 minutes, or until desired tenderness. Remove greens and press out excess water. Chop, mix in some lime juice, and season to taste. Set aside for later use.

For the fish: Heat the oil in a nonstick pan over medium heat. Add the fillets and brown. Turn over and cook for 2 minutes. Add a little lime juice, pepper, cover, and reduce heat. Cook the fillets until the flesh starts to flake. Transfer to a serving platter and cover with aluminum foil to keep warm. Add the onion, garlic, ginger, stock, remaining lime juice, honey, and rosemary to the pan. Mix well and bring to a boil. Reduce the sauce to end up with approximately 2/3 cup. Add a little cornstarch mixed with water to thicken the sauce. Strain and return to pan. Add the parsley and adjust seasonings. Pour over the fillets and serve immediately with the cooked greens.

nutritional facts

Per Serving: 329 Cal (23% from Fat, 53% from Protein, 24% from Carb); 42 g Protein; 8 g Tot Fat; 1 g Sat Fat; 4 g Mono Fat; 19 g Carb; 5 g Fiber; 8 g Sugar; 217 mg Calcium; 6 mg Iron; 585 mg Sodium; 58 mg Cholesterol

Herrings with Potatoes and Onions

serves 4

ingredients

Four 4-ounce herrings
1 teaspoon canola oil
2 teaspoons olive oil
1 large onion, sliced
(about 8 ounces)
4 small red potatoes
(about 3 ounces each)

1 tablespoon garlic cloves,
minced
1 bunch fresh parsley, minced
dash of white vinegar
Salt and pepper to taste

cooking instructions

Place the potatoes into a pan and cover with water. Add 1 teaspoon salt and bring to a boil over high heat. Reduce heat and simmer for 15 minutes. When barely cooked, strain and let cool a bit. Peel and slice the potatoes. Preheat the oven to 400 degrees F. Heat the canola oil in a nonstick pan over high heat. Add the onions and slightly brown. Add the garlic and continue to cook for 1 minute. Remove from heat and cool. Place each herring on a piece of aluminum foil. Open the herrings and sprinkle with a little pepper. Equally divide the potatoes and onions among the herrings. Sprinkle with olive oil and parsley. Close the foils tight and place in a baking dish. Bake for 25 to 30 minutes. Serve immediately with a dash of white vinegar.

nutritional facts

Per Serving (4 ounces herring):
471 Cal (34% from Fat, 27% from Protein, 39% from Carb); 32 g Protein; 18 g Tot Fat; 4 g Sat Fat; 8 g Mono Fat; 46 g Carb; 8 g Fiber; 4 g Sugar; 141 mg Calcium; 8 mg Iron; 1061 mg Sodium; 93 mg Cholesterol

Mackerel with Garlic and Steamed Vegetables

serves 4

ingredients

Four 5-ounce mackerels
16 garlic cloves, peeled
2 tablespoons olive oil
Salt and pepper to taste

For the vegetables:
4 large carrots, sliced
(about 1 pound)
3 large zucchini, sliced
(about 1 pound)
1 lemon, quartered
Salt and pepper to taste

cooking instructions

For the fish: Sprinkle pepper and a little salt inside the mackerels. Grease the bottom of a baking pan. Blanch the garlic cloves in boiling water for 3 minutes. Slightly crush them on the bottom of the greased pan. Top them with the mackerels and spread the remaining oil over the fish. Bake for 20 to 25 minutes.

For the vegetables: Preheat a steamer. Add the carrots and cook for 4 minutes. Add the zucchini and continue to cook for 2 to 3 minutes or until desired doneness. Transfer to a serving platter and season to taste. Serve the mackerels with the vegetables and lemon wedges.

nutritional facts

Per Serving (5 ounces mackerel):
436 Cal (54% from Fat, 27% from
Protein, 19% from Carb); 30 g Protein; 27 g Tot Fat; 6 g Sat Fat; 13 g
Mono Fat; 21 g Carb; 6 g Fiber; 7 g
Sugar; 107 mg Calcium; 3 mg Iron;
220 mg Sodium; 99 mg Cholesterol

Cioppino

serves 6

ingredients

1 tablespoon olive oil
1 small onion, julienned
(about 4 ounces)
1 medium green bell pepper, julienned (about 6 ounces)
1 small fennel bulb, julienned
(about 6 ounces)
4 garlic cloves, minced
5 plum tomatoes, peeled, seeded, and diced (about 1 pound)

1 tablespoon tomato paste
1 1/3 cup fish or vegetable stock
(low-fat and low-sodium)
Four 5 ounce fish steaks
(shark, halibut, or tuna)
1 bouquet garni
8 clams
8 mussels
8 shrimps, peeled and de-veined
1 bunch of basil, minced
Salt and pepper

cooking instructions

Make a small X incision on the top and bottom of the tomatoes. Blanch the tomatoes for 15 seconds. Remove and place in ice-cold water to stop the cooking process. Peel, seed, and chop the tomatoes.

Heat the oil in a pan over high heat. Add the onions, peppers, fennel, garlic, and sauté for 4 minutes. Add the diced tomatoes, tomato paste, and stir for a minute. Add the stock, fish, bouquet garni, and bring to a boil. Reduce heat and simmer for 5 minutes. Add clams, mussels, shrimps, and cook until the shells open. Remove bouquet garni, add basil, and adjust seasonings.

nutritional facts

Per Serving: 263 Cal (22% from Fat, 55% from Protein, 23% from Carb); 36 g Protein; 7 g Tot Fat; 1 g Sat Fat; 3 g Mono Fat; 15 g Carb; 3 g Fiber; 5 g Sugar; 142 mg Calcium; 6 mg Iron; 344 mg Sodium; 65 mg Cholesterol

Shrimp Scampi Style

serves 4

ingredients

4 tablespoons olive oil

2 pounds large shrimps, shelled and de-veined

2 medium red bell peppers; seeded, ribs removed, and sliced (about 12 ounces)

4 large garlic cloves, minced

1/2 lemon with its zest set aside

2 tablespoons freshly minced basil

1/2 cup whole wheat pasta

Salt and pepper to taste

cooking instructions

Cook the pasta according to package directions. Heat the oil and garlic in a large pan over medium heat. Add the shrimp and cook for 1 minute or until fully cooked, stirring occasionally. Add the bell peppers, lemon juice, lemon peel, basil, and season to taste. Continue to cook for 2 minutes or until the shrimp are cooked through, stirring occasionally. Add the cooked pasta and serve immediately.

nutritional facts

Per Serving: 496 Cal (32% from Fat, 41% from Protein, 26% from Carb); 52 g Protein; 18 g Tot Fat; 3 g Sat Fat; 11 g Mono Fat; 33 g Carb; 2 g Fiber; 4 g Sugar; 161 mg Calcium; 7 mg Iron; 343 mg Sodium; 345 mg Cholesterol

Scallops with Tangerines

serves 4

ingredients

1 tablespoon olive oil

1 pound scallops

6 tangerines

1 cup orange juice

1 teaspoon minced ginger

1 shallot, minced

8 ounces mushrooms

2 tablespoons parsley, minced

Olive oil

Salt and pepper

cooking instructions

Peel and segment the tangerines. Place the orange juice and half of the ginger in a saucepan and bring to a boil over high heat. Reduce until you end up with 1/4 cup and set aside.

Heat 1 teaspoon of olive oil in a saucepan over high heat. Add the mushrooms, shallot, remaining ginger, and sauté quickly. Add parsley and season to taste.

Meanwhile, lightly season the scallops. Heat 2 teaspoons of olive oil in a large saucepan over high heat. Add the scallops and sear on both sides. Add the mandarin segments, reduced orange juice, and continue to sauté for 1 minute. Serve immediately with the mushrooms and drizzle with a little olive oil.

nutritional facts

Per Serving: 241 Cal (18% from Fat, 36% from Protein, 46% from Carb); 22 g Protein; 5 g Tot Fat; 1 g Sat Fat; 3 g Mono Fat; 29 g Carb; 4 g Fiber; 19 g Sugar; 62 mg Calcium; 1 mg Iron; 189 mg Sodium; 37 mg Cholesterol

Meat/Poultry/Vegetable Entrées

It is important to your health to make sure you get the right amount of a good lean source of protein. You may already know that **animal protein is not as healthy for you as other, leaner protein sources** such as beans or tofu; this is because meat can raise cholesterol levels. Seek out organic meat and poultry (or free-range). This is healthier for you, due to the animal's natural diet, which results in higher amounts of beneficial fats such as Omega-3.

Here are some good general rules for selecting meat: **choose white meat such as chicken or turkey breast over darker meat.** Favor skinless pieces and, if cooking with the skin, avoid eating poultry cooked skin which is loaded with fat. Note that beef, lamb, mutton, and pork, which are higher in fat, should be eaten sparingly, and this is why this book features only a few recipes with these meats. When you do eat them, choose tender loin cuts. Choose buffalo or venison over beef. Avoid sausages, bacon, and pâtés due to their high unhealthy fat content. **Employ healthy cooking techniques such as baking, broiling, grilling, barbecuing, or sautéing in a nonstick pan with very little oil.** This limits the addition of fat and calories during preparation while preserving the succulent flavor of the meats.

Roasted Chicken Breast with Sweet Potatoes

serves 4

ingredients

2 tablespoons olive oil
1 teaspoon Italian seasoning
Four 4-ounce skinless
chicken breasts
4 sweet potatoes,
quartered (about 1 pound)

1 large yellow bell pepper,
chopped (about 8 ounces)
1 large zucchini, chopped
(about 8 ounces)

✓ *For a change: Yo*
may use different
herbs. You can also
sprinkle the potatoe.
with pumpkin pie
spices instead of her.
If so, place the potat
on one side of the pa
and the vegetables o
the other side.

cooking instructions

Preheat oven to 400ºF. In large bowl mix half of the oil with the chicken and transfer to a roasting pan. Toss the remaining oil with the sweet potatoes, bell pepper, and zucchini. Transfer to the roasting pan, arranging them around the chicken breasts. Sprinkle with the Italian herbs and season to taste. Roast until the chicken and vegetables are tender, about 25 to 30 minutes, turning them over halfway through the cooking time. Remove from the oven and serve immediately.

nutritional facts

Per Serving: 271 Cal (35% from Fat, 52% from Protein, 13% from Carb); 34 g Protein; 10 g Tot Fat; 2 g Sat Fat; 6 g Mono Fat; 9 g Carb; 2 g Fiber; 3 g Sugar; 43 mg Calcium; 2 mg Iron; 82 mg Sodium; 87 mg Cholesterol

Chicken Cacciatore

serves 6

ingredients

2 tablespoons olive oil
One 4-pound roasting chicken,
cut into serving pieces
1/4 cup chicken stock
(low-fat and low-sodium)
1 medium onion, diced
(about 6 ounces)
1 large carrot, diced
(about 4 ounces)
2 celery stalks, diced
(about 4 ounces)

1 medium green bell pepper,
diced (about 6 ounces)
2 garlic cloves, minced
1 cup canned diced tomatoes
1 cup mushrooms, sliced
Couple pinches of dry
Italian herbs
1/2 cup wild rice
Salt and pepper to taste

cooking instructions

Preheat the oven to 300°F. Heat a third of the oil in a large pan over high heat. Add half the chicken pieces and brown on all sides. Transfer to a large deep ovenproof pan and repeat the process with a third of the oil and remaining chicken pieces. Deglaze the pan with a little chicken stock and, with a whisk scrap all of the particles from the bottom and sides of the pan. Add liquid and particles to the chicken. Add remaining oil and slightly brown the onion.

Add the carrot, celery, garlic, tomatoes, mushrooms, herbs, and bring to a boil over medium heat. Season to taste and transfer to the chicken pan. Cover with aluminum foil and bake for 40 to 45 minutes.

Meanwhile, cook the wild rice according to package directions. Serve with the prepared chicken when done.

nutritional facts

Per Serving: 489 Cal (56% from Fat, 29% from Protein, 15% from Carb); 35 g Protein; 30 g Tot Fat; 8 g Sat Fat; 12 g Mono Fat; 19 g Carb; 3 g Fiber; 3 g Sugar; 48 mg Calcium; 3 mg Iron; 63 mg Sodium; 170 mg Cholesterol

Lemon Chicken

serves 4

> ✓ *This lemon chicken can also be used for appetizers, salads, soups, etc...*

ingredients

3 tablespoons olive oil
Four 4-ounce skinless chicken breasts
5 lemons
1 tablespoon fresh poultry herbs
Salt and pepper to taste

cooking instructions

Juice four lemons. Mix in two tablespoons of olive oil, the herbs, and season with pepper. Place the chicken pieces in a plastic bag. Pour the lemon marinade over the chicken and refrigerate for at least one hour, rotating every 10 minutes.

Preheat the broiler. Remove the chicken breasts from the marinade and pat dry. Place them on a greased cookie sheet and brush a little olive oil over each breast. Broil for approximately 6 to 7 minutes on each side. Watch carefully to avoid burning. Serve immediately with lemon wedges.

nutritional facts

Per Serving: 245 Cal (29% from Fat, 49% from Protein, 22% from Carb); 34 g Protein; 9 g Tot Fat; 1 g Sat Fat; 5 g Mono Fat; 15 g Carb; 6 g Fiber; 0 g Sugar; 107 mg Calcium; 2 mg Iron; 97 mg Sodium; 82 mg Cholesterol

Chicken Breast with Asian Glaze

serves 4

✓ *Suggestion: Serve with Swiss Chards Tagine (see page 113)*

ingredients

Four 5-ounce chicken breasts with bones and skin

2 tablespoons maple syrup

1 tablespoon green tea

1 tablespoon Oriental hot mustard

1 garlic clove, minced

2 tablespoons sesame seeds

1 teaspoon dried ginger

Salt and pepper to taste

Canola oil

cooking instructions

Preheat the oven to 350°F. Wash and pat dry the chicken breasts. Carefully pass your fingers between the meat and the skin to loosen up the skin without breaking it.

Heat the maple syrup, tea, mustard, garlic, and ginger in a saucepan over low heat until well blended. Season to taste and set aside. Lift up the chicken skin and brush the mixture over the chicken meat. Sprinkle with the sesame seeds and cover the breasts with the skin. Brush canola oil over the skin and roast for 30 minutes, or until cooked through. Remove skin before serving.

nutritional facts

Per Serving: 305 Cal (47% from Fat, 41% from Protein, 12% from Carb); 31 g Protein; 16 g Tot Fat; 4 g Sat Fat; 6 g Mono Fat; 9 g Carb; 1 g Fiber; 6 g Sugar; 75 mg Calcium; 2 mg Iron; 91 mg Sodium; 91 mg Cholesterol

Chicken Breast with Dijon Mustard

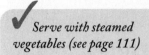

✓ *Serve with steamed vegetables (see page 111)*

serves 4

ingredients

Four 5-ounce skinless chicken breasts
1 tablespoon Dijon mustard
2 teaspoons lemon juice
1/2 teaspoon garlic powder
Canola oil
Salt and pepper to taste

cooking instructions

Preheat the oven to 375 °F. Place the chicken breasts in a lightly oiled pan. In a bowl, mix the mustard, lemon juice, and garlic powder. Spread over the chicken breasts and season to taste. Bake for 20 to 25 minutes, or until cooked through. Time may vary depending on the thickness of the breasts.

nutritional facts

Per Serving: 161 Cal (12% from Fat, 87% from Protein, 2% from Carb); 33 g Protein; 2 g Tot Fat; 0 g Sat Fat; 0 g Mono Fat; 1 g Carb; 0 g Fiber; 0 g Sugar; 19 mg Calcium; 1 mg Iron; 92 mg Sodium; 82 mg Cholesterol

Roasted Chicken Breast With Garlic Cloves

serves 4

✓ *Serve with steamed vegetables (see page 111) and lemon wedges.*

ingredients

Four 6-ounces chicken breasts
with bones and skin
8 to 10 garlic cloves
4 teaspoons olive oil
1 tablespoon dried Italian herbs
1 large lemon, cut in 8 slices

2 pinches of coarse salt
Pepper to taste

cooking instructions

Preheat the oven to 375 °F. Mince the garlic cloves on a clean cutting board. Sprinkle the coarse salt over the minced garlic cloves. Press with the side of a chef's knife until you end up with smooth paste. Transfer to a bowl. Mix in the olive oil, Italian herbs, and season with pepper. With your fingers, carefully separate the chicken skin slightly from the flesh, being careful not to break the skin. Spread the garlic mixture over the chicken flesh, add 2 lemon slices per breast, and push back the skin. Place the breasts in a baking dish and bake for 20 to 25 minutes, or until cooked through. Time may vary depending on the thickness of the breasts. Serve immediately and disregard skin when eating.

nutritional facts

Per Serving: 287 Cal (21% from Fat, 58% from Protein, 21% from Carb); 42 g Protein; 7 g Tot Fat; 1 g Sat Fat; 4 g Mono Fat; 15 g Carb; 2 g Fiber; 0 g Sugar; 114 mg Calcium; 3 mg Iron; 118 mg Sodium; 99 mg Cholesterol

Roasted Chicken Au Jus

serves 4 to 6

✔ *Suggestion: Serve with Potatoes Parsnip Purée (see page 116)*

ingredients

1 whole free-range organic chicken (4 pounds)

1 small onion, cut into 4 pieces (about 4 ounces)

1 medium carrot, cut into 4 pieces (about 3 ounces)

1 celery stalk, cut into 2 pieces

2 cups chicken stock (low-fat and low-sodium)

2 teaspoons dried thyme

2 teaspoons dried rosemary

Canola oil

Cornstarch with a little water

cooking instructions

Preheat the oven to 325 °F. Remove giblets from the chicken. Rinse chicken and pat dry. Season the inside of the chicken and add half of the herbs. Brush some oil over the chicken. Sprinkle with the remaining herbs and season to taste. Place the chicken in a roasting pan and roast for 2 to 2 ½ hours or until the juices come out clear. Remove the chicken from the pan and set aside covered to keep warm. Remove excess fat from the roasting pan. Add the vegetables, chicken stock, and deglaze the pan. Bring to a boil over medium heat and reduce to 1 cup. Strain, place in a saucepan, and add any rendered chicken juices. Bring to a boil and thicken with a little cornstarch water mixture. Serve immediately with the chicken.

nutritional facts

Per Serving: 286 Cal (60% from Fat, 32% from Protein, 8% from Carb); 22 g Protein; 19 g Tot Fat; 5 g Sat Fat; 7 g Mono Fat; 6 g Carb; 1 g Fiber; 2 g Sugar; 31 mg Calcium; 2 mg Iron; 299 mg Sodium; 106 mg Cholesterol

Cornish Hen with Olives

serves 4

ingredients

2 Cornish hens
1 tablespoon olive oil
3 large tomatoes (about 1 pound)
1 small onion, diced small
(about 4 ounces)
 3 garlic cloves, minced
6 ounces pitted green olives

3/4 cup chicken stock
(low-fat and low-sodium)
1/2 teaspoon Italian herbs
2 tablespoons fresh basil, minced
Salt and pepper to taste
1/2 cup brown rice

cooking instructions

Preheat the oven to 350 degrees F. Make a small X incision on the top
and bottom of the tomatoes. Blanch the tomatoes for 20 seconds. Place
in ice-cold water to stop the cooking process. Peel, seed, and dice the
tomatoes.

Wash and pat dry the inside and outside of the Cornish hens. Place the
hens in a baking pan, brush them with oil, and sprinkle with pepper.
Add the onion, tomatoes, garlic, 1/4 cup of stock, and mix in the herbs.
Bake for an hour. When the vegetables get too dry during the cooking
process, add more chicken stock.

Meanwhile, cook the rice according to package directions.

Remove the hens from the pan
and set aside in a serving platter.
Cover with aluminum foil to
keep warm. Transfer the sauce
to a saucepan. If the sauce is too
dry, add more chicken stock.
Add the olives, basil, and bring
to a boil. Pour the sauce over the
hens and serve immediately with
the brown rice.

nutritional facts

Per Serving: 490 Cal (60% from Fat,
26% from Protein, 14% from Carb);
31 g Protein; 32 g Tot Fat; 8 g Sat
Fat; 16 g Mono Fat; 17 g Carb; 3 g
Fiber; 1 g Sugar; 81 mg Calcium;
4 mg Iron; 521 mg Sodium;
170 mg Cholesterol

Chicken Burgers with Lettuce Wraps

✓ *Suggestion: Serve with Eggplant Mediterranean (see page 118)*

serves 2

ingredients

Four 4-ounce chicken burgers
4 garlic cloves, minced
4 tablespoons low-cal Caesar dressing
2 white anchovy fillet
16 lettuce leaves
4 tablespoons Parmesan Cheese
Canola oil
Salt and pepper to taste

cooking instructions

In a food processor puree the anchovy fillet with the dressing. Add a little water to thin out. Lightly season the burgers and shape them to fit in the lettuce leaves. Do not allow the meat to touch the leaves. Heat 2 tablespoons of olive oil with the minced garlic. Remove once boiling and set aside. Preheat the grill on medium high heat. Don't forget to grease the grill before adding the burgers. Cook them for 3 to 5 minutes on each side or until cooked through.

Meanwhile, carefully brush the garlic oil over the lettuce leaves.

nutritional facts

Per Serving: 381 Cal (49% from Fat, 42% from Protein, 9% from Carb); 40 g Protein; 20 g Tot Fat; 4 g Sat Fat; 12 g Mono Fat; 9 g Carb; 1 g Fiber; 3 g Sugar; 135 mg Calcium; 2 mg Iron; 429 mg Sodium; 104 mg Cholesterol (4 ounces chicken burger)

Place two leaves on a plate, top with one burger, spread 1 Tbsp. Caesar dressing, sprinkle with cheese and fold a bit over the top. Top with 2 more leaves and tuck underneath to seal. Serve immediately with your favorite accompaniment. You may use toothpick to hold for presentation.

Turkey Meatloaf with Tomato Sauce

serves 6

> ✓ *Suggestion: Serve with steamed vegetables such as broccoli and yellow squash.*

ingredients

1 teaspoon olive oil
1 small onion, minced
(about 4 ounces)
1 celery stalk, minced
(about 2 ounces)
2 garlic cloves, minced
1 pound ground buffalo meat
3/4 pound ground chicken or
turkey meat
3 ounces ground oats
1 large egg, beaten

3 ounces chicken stock
(low-fat and low-sodium)
1 teaspoon salt
1/4 teaspoon pepper
1/4 teaspoon dry mustard
1/8 teaspoon dry sage
1/2 teaspoon dry Italian herbs
10 ounces diced tomato

For serving: Your favorite tomato
sauce (about 1 cup)

cooking instructions

Preheat the oven to 350°F. Heat the oil in a pan over high heat.
Add the onion, celery, garlic, and cook for 2 minutes. Transfer
to a mixing bowl and add the remaining ingredients. Mix well
and place the meatloaf into a greased loaf pan. Bake the loaf for
1 hour to 1 ½ hour or until cooked through. Serve with your
favorite tomato sauce.

If buffalo meat is not available, substitute
with organic sirloin ground beef.

nutritional facts

Per Serving: 186 Cal (32% from Fat,
30% from Protein, 38% from Carb);
14 g Protein; 7 g Tot Fat; 2 g Sat
Fat; 2 g Mono Fat; 18 g Carb; 2 g
Fiber; 3 g Sugar; 50 mg Calcium;
2 mg Iron; 1123 mg Sodium;
69 mg Cholesterol

Turkey Breast with Italian Herbs

serves 8

> ✓ *Great way to prepare your own turkey breast meat for salads, snacks, soups, etc... You can also vary the flavoring by using different herbs. Sage is great and soothing.*

ingredients

1 tablespoon olive oil
2 pounds turkey breast
(with skin)
4 teaspoons Italian herbs
Bunch of fresh basil leaves
1/4 cup chicken stock
(low-fat and low-sodium)
Salt and pepper to taste

cooking instructions

Preheat the oven to 350° F. Mix 1 tablespoon of Italian herbs with a little pepper. Spread all over the turkey breast under its skin. Add as many basil leaves as you can fit under the skin without tearing the skin. Brush olive oil over the skin.

Place the turkey breast skin side up in a roasting pan. Pour 1/4 cup of chicken stock in the pan, add the remaining Italian herbs, and bake for an hour or until a meat thermometer registers 180° F. Keep moistening with chicken stock. To keep the turkey breast moist, do not allow the pan to get dry. Transfer the turkey breast to a platter and let cool before slicing.

nutritional facts

Per Serving: 199 Cal (46% from Fat, 52% from Protein, 2% from Carb); 25 g Protein; 10 g Tot Fat; 2 g Sat Fat; 4 g Mono Fat; 1 g Carb; 0 g Fiber; 0 g Sugar; 26 mg Calcium; 2 mg Iron; 119 mg Sodium; 74 mg Cholesterol

Stuffed Peppers

serves 4

✓ *You may substitute any type of cooked rice in this recipe.*

ingredients

1 teaspoon olive oil
4 large red bell peppers
1 small onion, diced
(about 4 ounces)
1 garlic clove, minced
3/4 pound ground turkey
1 cup cooked wild rice
3 tablespoons chopped parsley

2 pinches dry Italian herbs
1/4 cup chicken stock
(low-fat and low-sodium)
Salt and pepper
8 ounces tomato sauce

cooking instructions

Wash the peppers, cut off their tops, and remove their seeds and pith. Parboil the peppers 2 minutes in salted water. Remove the peppers from the pan and invert to drain over paper towels.

Heat the oil in a pan over medium heat. Add the onion, garlic, meat, and sauté until lightly browned. Add the wild rice, parsley, Italian herbs, stock, salt, pepper, and bring to a boil. Taste and adjust the seasonings. Cool down. Stuff the mixture inside the peppers and add the pre-cut tops.

Preheat the oven to 350°F. Place the peppers tightly into a greased pan, add a little water, and bake for 30 minutes. Heat the tomato sauce and serve with the cooked stuffed peppers.

nutritional facts

Per Serving: 281 Cal (20% from Fat, 41% from Protein, 39% from Carb); 29 g Protein; 6 g Tot Fat; 2 g Sat Fat; 2 g Mono Fat; 28 g Carb; 5 g Fiber; 8 g Sugar; 67 mg Calcium; 3 mg Iron; 450 mg Sodium; 65 mg Cholesterol

Turkey Chili

serves 4

ingredients

1 teaspoon canola oil
1 large onion, diced
(about 8 ounces)
1 medium green bell pepper;
cored, seeded, and diced
(about 6 ounces)
2 garlic cloves, minced
1 pound ground turkey
15 ounces canned diced tomatoes
2 ounces tomato paste

1 ¼ cup chicken stock
(low-fat and low-sodium)
12 ounces cooked kidney beans or
pinto beans
1 teaspoon dried thyme
1 teaspoon dried oregano
2 teaspoons ground cumin
2 tablespoons chili powder
1/4 teaspoon cayenne pepper
Salt to taste

cooking instructions

Heat the oil in a deep pan over medium heat. Add the meat and
brown slightly. Remove the excess fat rendered by the meat. Add
the onion, pepper, garlic, and mix well. Stir in the tomatoes, tomato
paste, stock, herbs, and spices. Bring to a boil and reduce heat.
Simmer uncovered for 30 to 40 minutes. Stir occasionally and
thicken longer, if necessary. Add the beans and bring to a simmer.
Adjust seasoning and serve immediately.

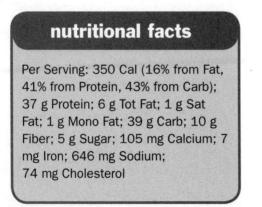

nutritional facts

Per Serving: 350 Cal (16% from Fat,
41% from Protein, 43% from Carb);
37 g Protein; 6 g Tot Fat; 1 g Sat
Fat; 1 g Mono Fat; 39 g Carb; 10 g
Fiber; 5 g Sugar; 105 mg Calcium; 7
mg Iron; 646 mg Sodium;
74 mg Cholesterol

Mediterranean Portobello Burger

serves 4

✓ *Suggestion: Combine with the Quinoa and Apricot Salad (see page 66) for a healthy meal.*

ingredients

4 teaspoons olive oil
4 large Portobello mushroom caps
2 garlic cloves, minced
4 onion slices
8 tomato slices
4 teaspoons feta cheese
4 tablespoons roasted red bell peppers spread

4 teaspoons black olives
8 large basil leaves
Bunch of lettuce leaves, wide enough to wrap the Portobello mushrooms
Cider vinegar
Salt and pepper to taste

cooking instructions

Preheat the grill on medium heat. Brush the Portobello mushrooms with olive oil and sprinkle them with pepper. Grill the mushroom caps for 2 minutes on each side. Grill the onion slices. Turn the mushrooms so that the top of the mushroom cap is on the grill. Now you can fill the inside cavity with the red bell pepper spread, garlic, olives, and season to taste. Grill for another minute or two.

Place each Portobello mushroom on a bunch of lettuce leaves (cap up-side down), add 1 tablespoon feta cheese, 1 grilled onion slice, 2 tomato slices, 2 basil leaves, and sprinkle with vinegar. Close the lettuce leaves to seal and serve immediately.

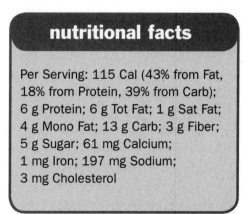

nutritional facts

Per Serving: 115 Cal (43% from Fat, 18% from Protein, 39% from Carb); 6 g Protein; 6 g Tot Fat; 1 g Sat Fat; 4 g Mono Fat; 13 g Carb; 3 g Fiber; 5 g Sugar; 61 mg Calcium; 1 mg Iron; 197 mg Sodium; 3 mg Cholesterol

Side Dishes & Snacks

Oftentimes, proteins are the focus of meals. However, you must not forget about the importance of side dishes and snacks. For one thing, their nutritional value can help complete a day's minimum requirements for fiber, vitamin and mineral intake. Once more, **carefully chosen snacks and side dishes keep us from becoming bored with food.** This is key, for it is often boredom that leads us to binge on poor food choices.

Side dishes should emphasize plenty of vegetables and include an appropriate amount of complex carbohydrates based on your daily activities. Emphasize whole grains rather than refined grains, as they contain antioxidants, lignans, and minerals which fight cancer and reduce oxidation in the body.

Always keep the fat content low in your snacks and side dishes. Snacks should also feature fresh food sources such as fruits, and vegetables high in calcium. Nuts are good too, as long as you are not allergic. Low-fat dairies (cottage cheese and yogurt) should also be a priority on your snacks list because they contain calcium, essential vitamins, and live bacterial cultures, which may help you live longer and may fortify your immune system. Purchase plain organic products with live cultures and no sugar added. Add fresh cut fruits, preserves, or honey to provide sweetness.

Vegetarian Chili

serves 4

ingredients

1 tablespoon canola oil or olive oil
2 medium onions, chopped (about 12 ounces)
2 garlic cloves, minced
1 large green bell pepper; cored, seeded, and diced
(about 8 ounces)
1 large red bell pepper; cored, seeded, and diced
(about 8 ounces)
1 large zucchini, diced
(about 8 ounces)
1 large yellow squash, diced
(about 8 ounces)

2 large Portobello mushrooms, diced
15 ounces canned diced tomatoes
1 1/2 cups vegetable stock (low-fat and low-sodium)
12 ounces corn kernels
3 cups cooked kidney beans or pinto beans
1 teaspoon dried thyme
1 teaspoon dried oregano
2 teaspoons ground cumin
2 tablespoons chili powder
1/4 teaspoon cayenne pepper
Salt to taste
Cornstarch with a little water

cooking instructions

Heat the oil in a deep pan over medium heat. Add the onions, garlic, and sauté for 2 minutes. Add the bell pepper, zucchini, yellow squash, mushrooms, diced tomatoes, stock, spices, herbs, and bring to a boil. Reduce heat and simmer until the vegetables are tender. Pass through a sieve and return the liquid to the pan. Reduce over high heat to concentrate the flavors and adjust seasoning. If needed, thicken with a little cornstarch water mixture. Return the vegetables to the reduced liquid and serve immediately.

nutritional facts

Per Serving: 432 Cal (14% from Fat, 19% from Protein, 67% from Carb); 22 g Protein; 7 g Tot Fat; 1 g Sat Fat; 3 g Mono Fat; 80 g Carb; 18 g Fiber; 14 g Sugar; 132 mg Calcium; 8 mg Iron; 416 mg Sodium; 0 mg Cholesterol

Steamed Vegetables

serves 4

ingredients

2 cups baby carrots
(about 8 ounces)
1 medium head broccoli
florets (about 8 ounces)
1/2 small head cauliflower florets
(about 8 ounces)

1 tablespoon fresh salad herbs
1 lemon, juiced
Salt and pepper to taste

cooking instructions

Steaming is a very fast cooking process, so pay attention since your vegetables can be overcooked very quickly. Cut the vegetables the same size for even cooking.

Mix the lemon juice, herbs, and set aside. Preheat a steamer. When the water is boiling, add the carrots and cauliflower florets in even layers to ensure uniform cooking. Cook covered for 4 minutes. Add the broccoli florets, cover, and cook for 1 to 2 minutes. Transfer the vegetables to a serving bowl. Mix in the lemon juice mixture, season to taste, and serve immediately.

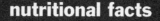

nutritional facts

Per Serving: 56 Cal (8% from Fat,
19% from Protein, 73% from Carb);
3 g Protein; 1 g Tot Fat; 0 g Sat Fat;
0 g Mono Fat; 13 g Carb; 6 g Fiber;
4 g Sugar; 76 mg Calcium;
1 mg Iron; 62 mg Sodium;
0 mg Cholesterol

Marinated Vegetables with Lemon

serves 4

ingredients

1 large onion (about 8 ounces)
2 large carrots (about 8 ounces)
8 asparagus (about 8 ounces)
1 medium head broccoli florets
(about 8 ounces)

For the marinade:
1 lemon
1 tablespoon garlic cloves,
minced

1 branch fresh thyme, minced
1 teaspoon honey
1 tablespoon rice vinegar
3 tablespoons olive oil
1 teaspoon dry parsley
Salt and pepper to taste

cooking instructions

For the marinade: Remove zest from the lemon, mince, and place in a bowl. Juice the lemon and add to the bowl. Blend in the remaining marinade ingredients and set aside.

For the vegetables: Cut the vegetables the same size for even cooking. Parboil the carrots for 2 minutes and place immediately in ice-cold water.

Place all the vegetables in a plastic bag, add the marinade, mix well, and refrigerate for a minimum of 4 hours.

Preheat the oven to 450 F. Transfer the vegetables and marinade to a baking pan. Bake for 20 to 25 minutes or until desired doneness.

nutritional facts

Per Serving: 178 Cal (48% from Fat, 9% from Protein, 43% from Carb); 4 g Protein; 11 g Tot Fat; 1 g Sat Fat; 8 g Mono Fat; 22 g Carb; 5 g Fiber; 8 g Sugar; 93 mg Calcium; 2 mg Iron; 59 mg Sodium; 0 mg Cholesterol

Swiss Chard Tagine

serves 4

ingredients

2 pounds Swiss chard
1 small onion, diced
(about 4 ounces)
2 tablespoons olive oil
1 tablespoon garlic cloves,
minced
Salt, pepper, and paprika

cooking instructions

Wash the Swiss chard and blanch in simmering salted
water for 2 minutes. Strain and press out excess water.
Let cool and chop.

Heat the oil in a nonstick pan over high heat. Add the
onion, garlic, and sauté for 2 minutes. Add the Swiss
chard and cook for 5 minutes, or until tender. Sprinkle
with salt, pepper, and paprika to taste. Mix well and
serve immediately

nutritional facts

Per Serving: 118 Cal (50% from Fat,
14% from Protein, 37% from Carb);
4 g Protein; 7 g Tot Fat; 1 g Sat Fat;
5 g Mono Fat; 12 g Carb; 4 g Fiber;
4 g Sugar; 126 mg Calcium;
4 mg Iron; 484 mg Sodium;
0 mg Cholesterol

Stuffed Bell Peppers

serves 4

ingredients

4 large red bell peppers
1 tablespoon olive oil
1 small onion, diced
(about 4 ounces)
2 garlic cloves, minced
1 large tomato (about 5 ounces)
10 ounces cooked wild rice

5 ounces vegetable stock
(low-sodium)
3 tablespoons fresh parsley,
minced
2 pinches dry Italian herbs,
minced
8 ounces tomato sauce
Salt and pepper to taste

cooking instructions

Make a small X incision on the top and bottom of the tomatoes. Blanch the tomatoes for 20 seconds. Place in ice-cold water to stop the cooking process. Peel, seed, and dice the tomatoes.

Wash the bell peppers and cut off their tops. Remove ribs and seeds. Parboil the bell peppers for 2 minutes. Remove the bell peppers from the pan and invert to drain over paper towels.

Heat the oil in a nonstick pan over high heat. Add the onion and sauté until translucent. Add the garlic, rice, tomato, parsley, Italian herbs, 3 ounces of stock, and bring to a boil. Season to taste and remove from heat. Cool completely before filling the bell peppers with this mixture. Finish by adding their pre-cut tops.

Preheat the oven to 350 degrees F. Place the stuffed bell peppers in a greased pan. Add the remaining stock to the pan and bake for 25 to 30 minutes. Heat the tomato sauce and serve immediately with the stuffed bell peppers.

nutritional facts

Per Serving: 200 Cal (21% from Fat, 10% from Protein, 70% from Carb); 5 g Protein; 5 g Tot Fat; 1 g Sat Fat; 3 g Mono Fat; 37 g Carb; 6 g Fiber; 12 g Sugar; 47 mg Calcium; 2 mg Iron; 328 mg Sodium; 0 mg Cholesterol

White Bean Stew

serves 8

ingredients

1 teaspoon olive oil
2 pounds dried white beans
1 medium onion, diced
(about 6 ounces)
1 medium carrot, diced
(about 3 ounces)
2 medium celery stalks, diced
(about 3 ounces)
2 tablespoons garlic cloves,
minced

15 ounces canned tomato purée
1 tablespoon flour
2 tablespoons fresh parsley,
minced
1 bouquet garni
4 cups chicken stock
(low-fat and low-sodium)
Salt and pepper to taste

cooking instructions

Place the beans in a large stockpot and add enough water to cover them.
Bring to a boil over high heat. Remove from heat and let stand covered
for 30 minutes. Drain the beans and rinse under cold water.

Heat the oil in a large pan over high heat. Add the onion, carrot, celery
stalks, garlic, and sauté for 2 minutes. Mix in the flour. Add the beans,
bouquet garni, and 4 cups of stock. If the beans are not covered, add
enough water to do so. Bring to a boil, reduce heat, and simmer covered
for 1 to 1 1/2 hours, or until tender. Add the tomato purée and bring to a
boil. Add parsley and season to
taste. If the mixture is too thin,
remove some beans, mash them,
and add them back to the stew.
Serve immediately.

nutritional facts

Per Serving: 461 Cal (5% from Fat,
24% from Protein, 71% from Carb);
29 g Protein; 3 g Tot Fat; 1 g Sat
Fat; 1 g Mono Fat; 84 g Carb; 19 g
Fiber; 8 g Sugar; 310 mg Calcium;
14 mg Iron; 461 mg Sodium;
1 mg Cholesterol

Potato Parsnip Purée

serves 4

ingredients

4 medium white potatoes
(about 1 1/2 pounds)
2 large garlic cloves, peeled
1 small parsnip (about 3 ounces)
1/4 cup low-fat milk
1/2 tablespoon fresh parsley,
minced

1/2 tablespoon fresh chives,
minced
2 teaspoons olive oil
Salt and pepper to taste

cooking instructions

Peel and quarter the potatoes and parsnip. Place them in a deep
pan and add enough cold water to cover them. Add the garlic
cloves, 1/4 teaspoon salt, and bring to a boil over high heat.
Cook until tender, about 20 to 25 minutes. Pass through a sieve,
keeping some of the cooking liquid, and purée with a potato
masher. Add low-fat milk, olive oil, and mix quickly. If too thick,
add a little cooking liquid to get to the right consistency. Mix in
the parsley, chives, and season to taste. Serve immediately.

nutritional facts

Per Serving: 158 Cal (12% from Fat,
9% from Protein, 79% from Carb);
4 g Protein; 2 g Tot Fat; 0 g Sat Fat;
1 g Mono Fat; 32 g Carb; 5 g Fiber;
4 g Sugar; 44 mg Calcium;
1 mg Iron; 20 mg Sodium;
1 mg Cholesterol

Wild Rice with Lentils

serves 4

ingredients

2/3 cup wild rice, rinsed
(about 4 ounces)
1 1/4 cup lentils, rinsed
(about 5 ounces)
1 large onion, diced
(about 8 ounces)
1 large garlic clove, minced

1 teaspoon olive oil
1/2 teaspoon ground cumin
1/2 teaspoon ground coriander
1/2 teaspoon paprika
1 tablespoon fresh parsley
Salt and pepper to taste

cooking instructions

Place the lentils in a pan and cover with water. Bring to a boil over high heat and simmer for 10 minutes. Strain and set aside.

Heat the oil in a large pan over high heat. Add the onion and sauté until translucent. Add the garlic, lentils, rice, seasonings, and 6 cups of water. Bring to a boil, reduce heat, cover, and simmer for 30 minutes. Adjust seasoning and remove from heat. Set aside covered for 5 minutes before serving.

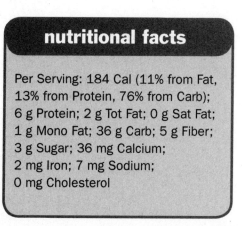

nutritional facts

Per Serving: 184 Cal (11% from Fat, 13% from Protein, 76% from Carb); 6 g Protein; 2 g Tot Fat; 0 g Sat Fat; 1 g Mono Fat; 36 g Carb; 5 g Fiber; 3 g Sugar; 36 mg Calcium; 2 mg Iron; 7 mg Sodium; 0 mg Cholesterol

Eggplant Mediterranean Style

serves 4

> ✓ *If ground thyme and oregano are difficult to find, use fresh versions and mince as small as possible.*

ingredients

2 small eggplants, both ends trimmed (about 1 pound)
2 tablespoons olive oil
1 teaspoon cumin
1 tablespoon paprika
1 tablespoon ground ginger
1 tablespoon garlic powder

1 teaspoon coriander
1/2 teaspoon cayenne pepper
1/4 teaspoon ground thyme
1/4 teaspoon ground oregano

cooking instructions

Cut eggplant slices lengthwise and arrange on baking sheet. Mix all the spices together. On both sides of the eggplant slices, brush olive oil, season with salt, and sprinkle the prepared spices. Preheat the broiler or barbecue. Broil or grill until golden brown, about 2 minutes per side.

nutritional facts

Per Serving: 199 Cal (61% from Fat, 6% from Protein, 33% from Carb); 3 g Protein; 15 g Tot Fat; 2 g Sat Fat; 10 g Mono Fat; 18 g Carb; 9 g Fiber; 6 g Sugar; 52 mg Calcium; 3 mg Iron; 10 mg Sodium; 0 mg Cholesterol

Sugar Snap Peas with Garlic

serves 4

ingredients

1 tablespoon olive oil
2 cups sugar snap peas
(about 8 ounces)
4 garlic cloves, sliced
1 lemon
Salt and pepper to taste

cooking instructions

Remove strings along both lengths of the sugar snap peas. Heat a wok with the olive oil over medium heat. Add the garlic and sauté quickly. Add the sugar snap peas and sauté until tender and crisp. Sprinkle with a little lemon juice, season to taste and serve immediately.

nutritional facts

Per Serving: 105 Cal (29% from Fat, 16% from Protein, 54% from Carb); 5 g Protein; 4 g Tot Fat; 1 g Sat Fat; 3 g Mono Fat; 16 g Carb; 5 g Fiber; 4 g Sugar; 47 mg Calcium; 1 mg Iron; 6 mg Sodium; 0 mg Cholesterol

Vegetables with Tapenade

serves 4

ingredients

3 ounces black olives, pitted
4 anchovy fillets, rinsed
and pat dry
3 teaspoons capers
1 small garlic clove
2 tablespoons olive oil

Lemon juice to taste
Pepper to taste
Vegetables such as carrots, bell
peppers, cherry tomatoes, and
mushrooms

cooking instructions

In a food processor purée the olives, anchovies, capers, and
garlic. Add pepper to taste. Slowly add the
olive oil until you obtain a smooth paste.
Add lemon juice to taste.

nutritional facts

Per Serving: 104 Cal (79% from Fat,
7% from Protein, 14% from Carb); 2
g Protein; 9 g Tot Fat; 1 g Sat Fat; 7
g Mono Fat; 4 g Carb; 1 g Fiber; 0
g Sugar; 42 mg Calcium; 1 mg Iron;
397 mg Sodium; 3 mg Cholesterol
(without vegetables)

Bell Peppers and Turkey Roll

serves 1

✓ *You may substitute eggplant spread with hummus. This may be served with a small salad on the side for a light lunch meal.*

ingredients

1/2 medium yellow squash, cut into strips (about 3 ounces)
1/2 medium bell pepper, seeded, ribs removed, and cut into strips (about 3 ounces)
1 tablespoon sun-dried tomatoes, minced

3 ounces turkey slices (about 1 ounce each or 3 slices)
3 tablespoons eggplant spread
6 basil leaves
Salt and pepper to taste

cooking instructions

Mix the sun-dried tomatoes and eggplant spread in a bowl. Lay each turkey slice on a large cutting board. Spread 1 tablespoon of the prepared mixture and 2 basil leaves over each turkey slice. Divide the bell pepper and zucchini strips equally on top of each turkey slice, and season to taste. Roll up each turkey slice and serve immediately.

nutritional facts

Per Serving: 180 Cal (31% from Fat, 34% from Protein, 34% from Carb); 17 g Protein; 7 g Tot Fat; 1 g Sat Fat; 1 g Mono Fat; 17 g Carb; 3 g Fiber; 7 g Sugar; 32 mg Calcium; 2 mg Iron; 1210 mg Sodium; 35 mg Cholesterol (3 turkey slices)

Wild Smoked Salmon Roll

serves 1

> ✔ *This may be served with a small salad on the side for a light lunch meal.*

ingredients

3 ounces smoked salmon
(about 4 slices)
12 asparagus, trimmed
(about 12 ounces asparagus)
4 tablespoons Boursin light
cheese
Pepper to taste

cooking instructions

Preheat a steamer over high heat. Add the asparagus, reduce heat, and cook until desired doneness. Remove from the steamer and blanch in ice-cold water to stop the cooking process.

Lay each smoked salmon slice on a large cutting board. Spread 1 tablespoon of Boursin over each slice. Add 3 asparagus per slice, sprinkle with pepper to taste, and roll. Serve immediately or refrigerate until needed.

nutritional facts

Per Serving: 264 Cal (33% from Fat, 45% from Protein, 22% from Carb); 31 g Protein; 10 g Tot Fat; 5 g Sat Fat; 2 g Mono Fat; 15 g Carb; 7 g Fiber; 6 g Sugar; 91 mg Calcium; 8 mg Iron; 986 mg Sodium; 32 mg Cholesterol

Radishes with Hazelnut Sour Cream

serves 4

✔ *Mix in a little horseradish or fine herbs. You may substitute low-fat sour cream with low-fat yogurt.*

ingredients

10 radishes
1 tablespoon low-fat sour cream
1 teaspoon low-fat milk
1 tablespoon hazelnuts
Pinch of salt
Pinch of pepper

cooking instructions

Crush and mince the hazelnuts with a chef knife. Mix the sour cream with the milk in a bowl. Add the minced hazelnuts, salt, and pepper. Serve immediately with the radishes.

nutritional facts

Per Serving: 79 Cal (63% from Fat, 12% from Protein, 24% from Carb); 3 g Protein; 6 g Tot Fat; 1 g Sat Fat; 4 g Mono Fat; 5 g Carb; 2 g Fiber; 3 g Sugar; 45 mg Calcium; 1 mg Iron; 58 mg Sodium; 4 mg Cholesterol

Apple and Almond Butter

serves 1

ingredients

1 small apple (about 4 ounces)
1 tablespoon almond butter

cooking instructions

Cut the apple in half, remove core, and slice. Equally spread
the almond butter among the slices.

nutritional facts

Per Serving: 153 Cal (51% from Fat,
6% from Protein, 43% from Carb); 3
g Protein; 9 g Tot Fat; 1 g Sat Fat; 6
g Mono Fat; 18 g Carb; 2 g Fiber; 11
g Sugar; 48 mg Calcium; 1 mg Iron;
2 mg Sodium; 0 mg Cholesterol

Cottage Cheese, Raisins, and Walnuts

serves 1

ingredients

1/3 cup low-fat cottage cheese,
cold
1 tablespoon chopped walnuts
2 teaspoons raisins
Cinnamon to taste

cooking instructions

Mix cottage cheese, walnut, and raisins. Sprinkle with
cinnamon to taste and serve immediately.

nutritional facts

Per Serving: 136 Cal (40% from Fat,
33% from Protein, 26% from Carb);
12 g Protein; 6 g Tot Fat; 1 g Sat
Fat; 1 g Mono Fat; 9 g Carb;
1 g Fiber; 5 g Sugar; 63 mg Calcium;
0 mg Iron; 307 mg Sodium;
6 mg Cholesterol

Sardines with Edamame

serves 2

ingredients

1 can sardines (about 4 ¼ ounces)
1/2 cup cooked Edamame
1/4 lemon, juiced
Salt and pepper to taste

cooking instructions

Roughly chop the sardines in a bowl. Mix in the Edamame and lemon juice. Season to taste and serve immediately.

nutritional facts

Per Serving: 192 Cal (44% from Fat, 39% from Protein, 17% from Carb); 19 g Protein; 10 g Tot Fat; 2 g Sat Fat; 3 g Mono Fat; 9 g Carb; 3 g Fiber; 0 g Sugar; 169 mg Calcium; 3 mg Iron; 64 mg Sodium; 36 mg Cholesterol

Desserts

Often associated with high calories, **desserts should be considered a treat.** One exception to the rule is fruits, which are powerful anti-oxidants and should be eaten every day. For that reason, fruits are the dessert focus of this book. **Give preference to berries, citrus, kiwis, and all yellow/orange/red/dark colored fruits.** However, be careful of possible allergies, particularly with strawberries, citrus, and kiwis. Whenever possible replace sugar with honey, maple syrup, or agave syrup. **A combination of organic plain low-fat dairy products and fruits** are also healthy dessert choices for providing calcium to your body.

Apple and Pear Minestrone

serves 2

ingredients

1 medium apple, brunoise
(about 5 ounces)
1 medium pear, brunoise
(about 5 ounces)
3/4 cup jasmine green tea
(or your favorite)
1 ½ teaspoon honey

1/2 teaspoon pumpkin pie spices
1 small ginger root, minced
1/2 teaspoon lemon zest
1/2 teaspoon grapeseed oil

cooking instructions

Heat the oil in a deep saucepan over high heat. Add the apple and
sauté for two minutes. Add the pear, spices, ginger, lemon zest,
and sauté another minute. Add the green tea and bring to a boil.
Remove from heat and transfer to a serving bowl. Cool at room
temperature. Refrigerate for an hour or, even better, overnight to
allow flavors to emerge. Serve cold.

nutritional facts

Per Serving: 105 Cal (10% from Fat,
2% from Protein, 88% from Carb); 1
g Protein; 1 g Tot Fat; 0 g Sat Fat; 0
g Mono Fat; 25 g Carb; 3 g Fiber; 18
g Sugar; 19 mg Calcium; 1 mg Iron;
2 mg Sodium; 0 mg Cholesterol

Baked Apples with Cranberries

serves 4
1 serving: 1 apple

ingredients

4 large apples
3 tablespoons red currant jelly
4 tablespoons cranberry juice
4 teaspoons walnuts
4 teaspoons cranberries

cooking instructions

Preheat the oven to 400 degrees F.

Wash and core the apples, being careful not to break through the bottom of the apples. Place them in a baking pan that is just the right size to keep the apples close to each other. Put 1 teaspoon of red currant jelly in the cavity of each apple. Pour one tablespoon of cranberry juice over the cavity of each apple. Add a little hot water in the pan (1/4 inch). Cover the pan with aluminum foil and bake for 20 minutes. Remove cover and baste with the liquid in the pan. Continue baking uncovered for 4 to 5 minutes. If necessary, add a little more water to avoid burning.

Place each apple in a serving dish. Scrape particles from the pan and transfer the liquid to a saucepan. Blend the liquid with the remaining red currant jelly and bring to a boil over high heat. Pour over the apples, sprinkle with the walnuts, cranberries, and serve immediately.

nutritional facts

Per Serving: 162 Cal (10% from Fat, 2% from Protein, 88% from Carb); 1 g Protein; 2 g Tot Fat; 0 g Sat Fat; 0 g Mono Fat; 38 g Carb; 5 g Fiber; 27 g Sugar; 17 mg Calcium; 0 mg Iron; 7 mg Sodium; 0 mg Cholesterol

Acai and Almond Milk Popsicle

✓ *Option: You may substitute almond milk with soy milk or low-fat milk.*

serves 4

ingredients

3.5 ounces Pure Acai, no sugar
added (Sambazon smoothie pack)
4 ounces berries (about 1 cup)
1 small banana (about 4 ounces)
4 ounces almond milk

cooking instructions

Place all the fruits and almond milk in a blender. Purée on high speed. Divide equally among 4 popsicles maker and freeze.

nutritional facts

Per Serving (1 popsicle): 68 Cal (25% from Fat, 11% from Protein, 64% from Carb); 2 g Protein; 2 g Tot Fat; 0 g Sat Fat; 0 g Mono Fat; 13 g Carb; 3 g Fiber; 6 g Sugar; 35 mg Calcium; 0 mg Iron; 20 mg Sodium; 0 mg Cholesterol

Red Fruits Compote

serves 4

✓ *Suggestion: Serve with low-fat yogurt, sherbet, cream of millet, apple slices, etc…*

ingredients

8 ounces blackberries
8 ounces raspberries
8 ounces blueberries
8 ounces strawberries
3 tablespoons honey

1 large organic lemon peel
1 large organic orange peel
1 cup pomegranate juice
(no sugar added)
Cornstarch and water

cooking instructions

Wash the berries and carefully pat dry. Place the pomegranate juice in a saucepan and bring to boil over high heat. Reduce by half. If necessary, thicken with a little water-cornstarch mixture. Add the honey, berries, and cook for a minute or two. Do not overcook, or you will end up with a sauce rather than a compote. Remove from heat and transfer the compote to a bowl. Place the bowl in an ice-cold water bath to stop the cooking process. Refrigerate for two hours before serving.

nutritional facts

Per Serving: 166 Cal (4% from Fat, 4% from Protein, 91% from Carb); 2 g Protein; 1 g Tot Fat; 0 g Sat Fat; 0 g Mono Fat; 42 g Carb; 8 g Fiber; 32 g Sugar; 37 mg Calcium; 1 mg Iron; 3 mg Sodium; 0 mg Cholesterol

Grilled Mango and Almonds

serves 4

ingredients

4 mangos, slightly firm, peeled
and thickly sliced
4 tablespoons sliced almonds
4 teaspoons honey
1 orange, juiced

cooking instructions

Preheat the broiler. Cover the bottom of a baking sheet with
parchment paper. Add the sliced almonds and broil until
slightly browned. Remove the almonds from the sheet and
cool.

Cover the bottom of a baking sheet with parchment paper.
Add the mango slices and broil until slightly browned.
Meanwhile heat the honey with the orange juice in a pan and
bring to a boil. Divide the mango slices among four plates.
Drizzle with the warm sauce, sprinkle
with the sliced almonds, and serve
immediately.

nutritional facts

Per Serving (1 mango): 207 Cal
(14% from Fat, 5% from Protein,
81% from Carb); 3 g Protein; 4 g Tot
Fat; 0 g Sat Fat; 2 g Mono Fat; 47 g
Carb; 5 g Fiber; 40 g Sugar; 51 mg
Calcium; 1 mg Iron; 5 mg Sodium;
0 mg Cholesterol

Papaya Brulée

serves 2

ingredients

2 small papayas
4 teaspoons brown sugar

cooking instructions

Preheat the broiler. Cut the papayas in half and remove
the seeds. Spread the sugar over each half. Place under the
broiler and grill until caramelized. This is pretty quick, so
keep an eye on the papayas. It will take approximately
1 minute.

nutritional facts

Per Serving: 145 Cal (2% from Fat,
4% from Protein, 93% from Carb);
2 g Protein; 0 g Tot Fat; 0 g Sat Fat;
0 g Mono Fat; 37 g Carb; 5 g Fiber;
26 g Sugar; 76 mg Calcium;
0 mg Iron; 12 mg Sodium;
0 mg Cholesterol

Peach with Apricot Coulis

serves 4

ingredients

4 peaches
12 apricots
1 tablespoon honey
1 teaspoon lemon juice
1 rosemary branch
4 teaspoons almonds

cooking instructions

Cut apricots in half and remove pits. Place the apricots in a pan.
Add 1/2 cup water, honey, rosemary, lemon juice, and bring to a
boil. Reduce heat, cover, and simmer for ten minutes. Purée in a
blender and transfer to a serving bowl. Let cool and refrigerate.
Peel and cut the peaches in half. Place the peach halves in
a serving platter, drizzle with some apricot sauce and the
almonds. Serve with the remaining apricot sauce on the side.

nutritional facts

Per Serving: 112 Cal (11% from Fat,
8% from Protein, 80% from Carb);
3 g Protein; 2 g Tot Fat; 0 g Sat Fat;
1 g Mono Fat; 25 g Carb; 4 g Fiber;
22 g Sugar; 21 mg Calcium;
1 mg Iron; 1 mg Sodium;
0 mg Cholesterol

Strawberries and Spinach Smoothie

serves 2

ingredients

2 cups strawberries
(about 10 ounces)
1 bunch fresh spinach
1 banana
1 tablespoon flaxseeds
Aged balsamic vinegar to taste
(optional)
Ice cubes

cooking instructions

Place strawberries, spinach, and banana in a blender. Puree and mix in the aged balsamic vinegar (optional). Serve immediately.

nutritional facts

Per Serving: 178 Cal (13% from Fat, 15% from Protein, 72% from Carb); 8 g Protein; 3 g Tot Fat; 0 g Sat Fat; 0 g Mono Fat; 37 g Carb; 10 g Fiber; 17 g Sugar; 206 mg Calcium; 6 mg Iron; 138 mg Sodium; 0 mg Cholesterol

Spring Fruit Salad with White Tea

serves 4

ingredients

1 small banana, sliced
3 ounces strawberries, halved
3 ounces blueberries
3 ounces raspberries
1 small apple, cubed
2 large plums, quartered
1 white tea sachet
1 tablespoon honey
1 tablespoon lemon juice

cooking instructions

Boil 3/4 cup of water. Add the lemon juice, tea sachet, honey, and infuse until desired strength. Remove sachet and cool completely. Blend all the fruits in a large bowl. Add the cold tea and refrigerate for 30 minutes, mixing every 10 minutes. Serve cold.

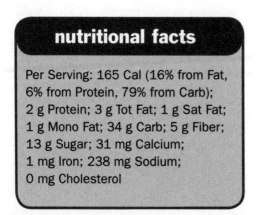

nutritional facts

Per Serving: 165 Cal (16% from Fat,
6% from Protein, 79% from Carb);
2 g Protein; 3 g Tot Fat; 1 g Sat Fat;
1 g Mono Fat; 34 g Carb; 5 g Fiber;
13 g Sugar; 31 mg Calcium;
1 mg Iron; 238 mg Sodium;
0 mg Cholesterol

Winter Fruit Salad

serves 4

ingredients

1 small banana, sliced
1 pear, diced
1 apple, diced
6 ounces grapes
1 orange, peeled and segmented
1/4 cup pomegranate seeds
2 tablespoons lemon juice

cooking instructions

Blend all the fruits in a large bowl. Mix in the lemon juice, pomegranate seeds, and refrigerate until use.

nutritional facts

Per Serving: 135 Cal (2% from Fat, 4% from Protein, 94% from Carb); 1 g Protein; 0 g Tot Fat; 0 g Sat Fat; 0 g Mono Fat; 35 g Carb; 4 g Fiber; 25 g Sugar; 31 mg Calcium; 0 mg Iron; 3 mg Sodium; 0 mg Cholesterol

Melon Soup

serves 4

ingredients

2 cantaloupes (or 4 cups)
2 tablespoons honey (quickly
warmed in the microwave)
4 mint leaves
1 lemon, juiced

cooking instructions

Cut the cantaloupes in half. Remove seeds. Spoon out
the flesh and place in a blender. Add the honey, mint, and
lemon juice. Purée and
refrigerate. Serve cold.

nutritional facts

Per Serving: 98 Cal (3% from Fat,
6% from Protein, 90% from Carb);
2 g Protein; 0 g Tot Fat; 0 g Sat Fat;
0 g Mono Fat; 26 g Carb; 3 g Fiber;
23 g Sugar; 33 mg Calcium;
1 mg Iron; 30 mg Sodium;
0 mg Cholesterol

Thin Peach and Apricot Tart

serves 8

ingredients

3 ounces almond meal

2 ounces oats

3 tablespoons grapeseed oil

Pinch of salt

1 tablespoon almond extract

2 to 3 tablespoons ice cold water

2 tablespoons apricot preserves

2 large peaches (about 8 ounces)

4 large apricots (about 8 ounces)

cooking instructions

Preheat the oven to 475°F. Place the oats in a blender and reduce to a flour consistency. Place the oat and almond flours in a bowl. Add salt, oil, almond extract, and mix until crumbly. Add one tablespoon water at a time and continue until the dough is smooth and sticks together as one ball. Lay the dough on wax paper and push down with your palm to flatten a bit. Roll out the dough to a round thin form. Then turn over the dough to a cookie sheet. Brush 1 tablespoon preserves all over the pie dough surface. Peel the peaches, apricots, and cut in half. Core, quarter, and slice. Starting at the edge of the dough and working inward toward the center, arrange the peach slices in overlapping circles. Finish with a circle of apricot slices in the center. Bake for 15 to 20 minutes until golden brown with slightly darker edges. Heat the remaining preserves in the microwave with a little water to thin. Remove the tart from the oven and brush with the peach preserves. Transfer to a cooling rack.

nutritional facts

Per Serving: 177 Cal (55% from Fat, 9% from Protein, 36% from Carb); 4 g Protein; 11 g Tot Fat; 1 g Sat Fat; 1 g Mono Fat; 16 g Carb; 3 g Fiber; 8 g Sugar; 33 mg Calcium; 1 mg Iron; 5 mg Sodium; 0 mg Cholesterol

APPENDIX A

Meal Diary and Sample Menu

Meal Diary

Create a journal that you will complete every day to track your eating habits. No worries, you won't have to do this all your life. It might take you a while to figure things out, but eventually you will no longer need to write things down. You may include the following columns:

Date	Time	Food	Drink	Mood/ Pain level	Where you ate	Calories

An eating journal allows you to learn a lot about your own eating habits. It may help you to discover what you are doing wrong and to make appropriate adjustments on your own. You will be in a better position to design your own personal healthy eating habits and meals. You also will be able to provide great information to your medical provider who, in turn, will be in a better position to help you.

Here are a few examples of what you may observe by keeping a journal:
- You ate the wrong foods when you are stressed, at work, or at parties.
- You ate 500 calories over your daily allowances
- You ate a food which is on your allergy list
- Instead of eating a healthy breakfast, you just grab a cup of coffee and go

- You ate out and got sick afterwards
- You are skipping meals

What you find out may surprise you. This awareness of your habits will lead to positive changes. One simple change can make a huge difference in your well-being. Don't be overwhelmed, just look at your journal with objectivity and start to see where you can make a change. Start with one thing. Once you do, and feel great about the result, move on to the next one, and so on.

Sample Menus

The following menus have been designed to show you how you can plan and vary your meals while still staying within your recommended daily calories. Please feel free to adjust them to your preferences. Most of the recipes are based on the right amount of healthy fat, so you don't really have to worry about the amount. Feel free to use smaller portions of soups, salads, or vegetables recipes for snacks. If you need to lose weight, remember to consult your physician or registered dietitian. Discuss what is appropriate for your personal situation. Do not guess on your own, or you can jeopardize your health.

Meal	Recipe	Yield	Calories
Breakfast	All-Bran with Apples and Cinnamon (page 40)	1 serving	252
Lunch	Salmon with Orange Sauce (page 79)	1 serving	461
Snack	Beets with Shaved Pecorino (page 63)	1 serving	181
Dinner	Chicken Breast with Asian Glaze (page 97) Swiss chard Tagine (page 113)	1 serving 1 serving	305 118
Dessert	Peach with Apricot Coulis (page 134)	1 serving	112
Total calories			1429

Meal	Recipe	Yield	Calories
Breakfast	Cream of Millet (page 41)	1 serving	384
Snack	Bell Pepper and Turkey Roll (page 121)	1 serving	180
Lunch	Greek Salad with Cod Fish (page 65)	1 serving	222
Snack	Radish with Hazelnut Sour Cream (page 123)	1 serving	79
Dinner	Chicken Cacciatore (page 95)	1 serving	489
Dessert	Papaya Brulée (page 133)	1 serving	145
Total calories			1499

APPENDIX B

Substitutions

Sometimes it may be hard to find certain ingredients. What if you just ran out of one ingredient while preparing a dish, you are allergic to one ingredient and need a substitution, or you want to reduce the calories of a recipe? The following substitution list will be very useful during those times. Use simple judgment to choose the right substitution, depending on the application. Keep in mind every ingredient has a specific function in a recipe and making substitutions may alter the recipe. Baking is particularly a concern since it is all about chemistry. You may have to try a recipe many times before finding the right balance. Bes sure to take notes so you can remember what you did, especially when it turns out great!

Substitution List

1 tsp. allspice	½ tsp. cinnamon, ½ tsp. ground cloves, and ¼ tsp. nutmeg
1 tsp. baking powder	¼ tsp. baking soda plus ½ tsp. cream of tartar
1 cup butter	a little less than a cup of oil
1 cup buttermilk	1 cup plain yogurt Or 1 cup milk plus 1 Tbsp. lemon juice or vinegar Or 1 cup milk plus 1¾ tsp. cream of tartar
1 cup ketchup	1 cup tomato sauce, ½ cup sugar, and 2 Tbsp. vinegar
1 cup chili sauce	1 cup tomato sauce, ¼ cup brown sugar, 2 Tbsp. vinegar, ¼ tsp. cinnamon, dash of ground cloves, and dash of allspice.

1 oz. unsweetened chocolate	3 Tbsp. Carob powder plus 2 Tbsp. Water
1 cup cream cheese	1 cup part skim milk ricotta cheese or low-fat cottage cheese mixed until smooth or 1 cup of creamy or soft tofu plus a little lemon juice.
1 cup half-and-half cream	1 cup evaporated milk
1 cup cream	1 cup evaporated milk
1 cup heavy cream	2/3 cup buttermilk plus 1/3 cup oil or ½ cup part-skim milk ricotta cheese plus ½ cup nonfat yogurt
1 cup heavy cream will give 2 cups once whipped.	In some recipes, substitute 1 cup of creamy or soft tofu plus a little lemon juice. Replace 1 cup of whipped cream with 1 cup of evaporated nonfat milk placed in the freezer until icy and then whipped with a little vanilla powder. This is not very stable; use, as an example, to accompany fruit salad.
½ tsp. cream of tartar	1½ tsp. lemon juice or vinegar
1 large egg	2 egg whites
1 Tbsp. flour (for thickening purposes in cooking only)	1½ tsp. cornstarch or potato starch Or 1 Tbsp. sweet rice flour Or 1½ Tbsp. rice flour Or 1½ Tbsp. granular tapioca Or 2 tsp. quick-cooking tapioca Or 1½ tsp. Agar Or 3 tsp. bean flour Or 1½ tsp. Guar Gum Or 1 tsp. Xanthan Gum
1 cup all purpose flour (for cooking and not baking)	Or 1 cup tapioca flour Or ½ cup soy flour plus ½ cup potato starch flour Or ¾ cup cornstarch Or ¾ cup garbanzo flour Or ½ cup nut flour Or 7/8 cup rice flour Or 7/8 sorghum flour (Milo) Or 1¼ cup rye flour Or 1½ cup oat flour Or 1 cup corn flour Or ¾ cup coarse cornmeal ¾ cup potato starch flour

When baking, these substitutions do not necessary work well by themselves. Usually other ingredients from the recipe need adjustment. Unless you have a lot of time on your hands for trial and error, do not attempt to create baking recipes but rather use those already available in cookbooks in specialty stores or over the Internet.

1 Garlic clove	1/8 tsp. garlic powder
1 Tbsp. fresh grated ginger	1/8 tsp. powdered ginger
1 Tbsp. fresh herb	1 tsp. dry herb
1 tsp. lemon juice	½ tsp. vinegar
1 cup mayonnaise	½ cup yogurt plus ½ cup mayonnaise (canola preferably) Or 1 cup salad dressing such as vinaigrette Or 1 cup low-fat sour cream Or 1 cup low-fat yogurt Or 1 cup low-fat cottage cheese pureed in a blender until smooth
1 cup milk	½ cup evaporated milk plus ½ cup water Or 1 cup buttermilk plus ½ tsp. baking soda (for baking decrease baking powder by 2 tsp.) Or 4 Tbsp. whole dry milk plus 1 cup water Or 1cup other liquid
1-cup molasses	1 cup honey
1 Tbsp. prepared mustard	1 tsp. dry mustard plus 2 tsp. vinegar
Oats	Old-fashioned rolled oats and quick oats are interchangeable.
1 cup uncooked rice or pasta	3 cups cooked
A couple shreds of saffron	dash of turmeric mostly for color, but not quite the same flavor
1 cup sour cream	1/3 cup buttermilk plus 1 Tbsp. lemon juice plus 1 cup cottage cheese blended Or 1 cup low-fat yogurt Or 1 cup cottage cheese plus 2 tsp. lemon juice blended

1 cup granulated sugar	1 cup light brown sugar Or ½ cup molasses (reduce liquid in recipe by ¼ cup) Or ¾ cup honey (reduce liquid in recipe by ¼ cup and add ¼ tsp. baking soda) Reduce oven by 25° F when baking Or ¾ cup maple syrup (reduce liquid in recipe by ¼ cup and add ¼ tsp. baking soda), Or ¾ cup fruit juice concentrate (reduce liquid in recipe by 1/3 cup and add ¼ tsp. baking soda) Reduce oven by 25° F when baking. Or substitute only ½ of the sugar with ½ cup fruit puree Or 1 cup granulated fructose Or 1 cup liquid fructose. Reduce liquid in recipe by ¼ cup.
1 cup tomato juice	½ cup tomato sauce plus ½ cup water or vegetable stock
1 15 oz. can of tomato sauce	1 6 oz can of tomato paste plus 1 cup water
1 cup tomato soup	1 cup tomato sauce plus ¼ cup water or vegetable stock
1 tsp. vanilla extract	1 vanilla bean split and simmered in liquid from recipe
1 cup wine	1 cup stock
1 Tbsp. active dry yeast	1 cake compressed yeast or 1 package active dry yeast
1 cup plain yogurt	1 cup buttermilk Or 1 cup cottage cheese blended until smooth Or 1 cup low-fat sour cream Or 1 cup low-fat goat yogurt Or 1 cup low-fat soy yogurt

APPENDIX C

References and Resources

References

Dunne, Lavon J., *Nutrition Almanac,* Fifth Edition. McGraw Hill Companies, 2001.

Fenster, Carol. *Special Diet Solutions, Third Edition.* Savory Palate, Inc, 2001.

Lorig, Kate and David Sobel, *Living a Healthy Life with Chronic Conditions.* Bull Publishing Company, 2006.

Pappa, Apostolos and Marie-Annick Courtier, *The Saint-Tropez Diet.* Hatherleigh Press, 2007.

Sawyer, Ann D. and Judith E. Bachrach, *The MS Recovery Diet.* Penguin Books Ltd., 2007.

Swank, Laver Roy and Barbara Brewer Dugan, *The Multiple Sclerosis Diet* Book. Doubleday Publishing, 1987.

Resources

American Diabetes Association
ATTN: National Call Center
1701 North Beauregard StreetAlexandria, VA 22311
800-DIABETES (1-800-342-2383)
www.diabetes.org

American Dietetic Association
120 South Riverside Plaza
Suite 2000Chicago, IL 60606
800-877-1600
www.eatright.org

American Heart Association
7272 Greenville AvenueDallas, TX 75231
800-AHA-USA-1 (800-242-8721)
www.americanheart.org

Multiple Sclerosis Association of America
706 Haddonfield RoadCherry Hill, NJ 08002
800-532-7667
www.msassociation.org

National Multiple Sclerosis Society
800-344-4867
www.nationalmssociety.org